Clinical Electrocardiography

A Simplified Approach

Clinical Electrocardiography

A Simplified Approach

Ary L. Goldberger, M.D., F.A.C.C.

Associate Professor of Medicine, Harvard Medical School
Director of Electrocardiography, Beth Israel Deaconess Medical Center
Boston, Massachusetts

Sixth Edition

St. Louis   Baltimore   Boston   Carlsbad   Chicago   Minneapolis   New York   Philadelphia   Portland
London   Milan   Sydney   Tokyo   Toronto

Mosby
Dedicated to Publishing Excellence

A Times Mirror Company

Publisher: Laura DeYoung
Acquisitions Editor: Gina Almond
Developmental Editors: Beverly J. Copland and Pui Szeto
Project Manager: Linda McKinley
Production Editor: Barrett Schroeder
Design: Reneé Duenow
Cover Design: AKA Design Inc.
Manufacturing Manager: David Graybill

SIXTH EDITION
Copyright © 1999 by Mosby, Inc.

Printed in the United States of America
Composition by Graphic World
Printing/binding by Maple-Vail Book Manufacturing

Mosby, Inc.
11830 Westline Industrial Drive
St. Louis, Missouri 63146

Library of Congress Cataloging in Publication Data

Goldberger, Ary Louis, 1949–
    Clinical electrocardiography : a simplified approach / Ary L.
    Goldberger. — 6th ed.
        p.   cm.
    Includes bibliographical references and index.
    ISBN 0-323-00252-8
    1. Electrocardiography.   I. Title.
    [DNLM: 1. Electrocardiography.   WG 140 G616c 1999]
    RC683.5.E5G593   1999
    616.1'207547—dc21
    DNLM/DLC
    for Library of Congress   98-4102
                                                            CIP

98   99   00   01   02   /   9   8   7   6   5   4   3   2   1

For

Ellen, Zach, and Lexy

with love

Preface

This book is an introduction to electrocardiography. It is written particularly for medical students, house officers, and nurses, and it assumes no previous instruction in ECG reading. The book has been widely used in introductory courses on the subject. Clinicians wishing to review basic electrocardiography have also found it useful.

The book is divided into three sections. Part 1 covers the basic principles of electrocardiography, normal ECG patterns, and the major abnormal P-QRS-T patterns. Part 2 describes the major abnormalities of heart rhythm and conduction. Part 3 is a set of unknowns for review and self-assessment. In addition, practice questions are presented at the end of almost all chapters. In reading ECGs, as in learning a new language, fluency is attained only with repetition and review.

The clinical applications of ECG reading have been stressed throughout the book. Each time an abnormal pattern is mentioned, the conditions that might have produced it are discussed. Although the book is not intended to be a manual of therapeutics, general principles of treatment and clinical management are briefly discussed. Separate chapters are devoted to important special topics, including digitalis toxicity, cardiac arrest, the limitations and uses of the ECG, and pacemakers.

In addition, students are encouraged to approach ECGs in terms of a rational simple differential diagnosis, rather than through the tedium of rote memorization. It is comforting for most students to discover that the number of possible arrhythmias that can produce a heart rate of 170 beats per minute is limited to just a handful of choices. Only three basic ECG patterns are found with cardiac arrest. Similarly, only a few conditions cause low-voltage patterns, abnormally wide QRS complexes, etc.

In approaching any given ECG, three essential questions must always be addressed: What does the ECG show? What are the possible causes of this pattern? What, if anything, should be done about it? Most conventional ECG books focus on the first question, emphasizing pattern recognition. However, waveform analysis is only a first step, for example, in the clinical diagnosis of atrial fibrillation. The following questions must then be considered: What could have caused the arrhythmia, and what adverse effects might follow it? Treatment, of course, depends in part on the answers to these questions.

The aim of this book, therefore, is to present the ECG as it is used in hospital wards, outpatient clinics, emergency rooms, and intensive care units, where recognition of normal and abnormal patterns is only the starting point in patient care.

The sixth edition contains updated discussions on multiple topics, including arrhythmias and conduction disturbances, cardiac arrest and sudden death, myocardial ischemia and infarction, drug toxicity, and pacemakers. Differential diagnosis is highlighted, as are common pitfalls in ECG interpretation. Furthermore, the review questions throughout the text have been revised and updated. Part 3, a revamped self-assessment section, presents 50 ECG unknowns (with answers) at an intermediate to more advanced level.

This new edition is dedicated to the memory of my father, Emanuel Goldberger, M.D., a pioneer in the development of electrocardiography and the inventor of the aV_R, aV_L, and aV_F leads. He was the co-author of the previous editions of this textbook.

Ary L. Goldberger

Contents

Clinical Electrocardiography

A Simplified Approach

Part One

Basic Principles and Patterns

Introductory Principles

*T*he *electrocardiogram* (*ECG* or *EKG*) is a graphi-cal recording of the electrical activity of the heart. The ECG records cardiac electrical currents (voltages, potentials) by means of metal *electrodes* placed on the surface of the body.* As described in Chapter 3, these metal electrodes are placed on the arms, legs, and chest wall (precordium).

Basic Cardiac Electrophysiology

Before the basic ECG patterns are discussed, some elementary aspects of cardiac electrophysiology must be reviewed. Fortunately, only certain sim-ple principles are required for clinical interpreta-tion of ECGs.

The function of the heart is to contract rhyth-mically and pump blood to the lungs for oxy-genation and then to pump this oxygenated blood into the general (systemic) circulation. The signal for cardiac contraction is the spread of elec-trical currents through the heart muscle. These currents are produced both by pacemaker cells and specialized conducting tissue within the heart and by the heart muscle itself. The ECG records only the currents produced by the work-ing heart muscle.

ELECTRICAL STIMULATION OF THE HEART

The electrical "wiring" of the heart is outlined in Fig. 1.1. Normally the signal for cardiac electrical stimulation starts in the *sinus node,* also called the *sinoatrial* (SA) *node.* This node is located in the right atrium near the opening of the superior

vena cava. It is a small collection of specialized cells capable of automatically generating an elec-trical stimulus (signal). From the sinus node this stimulus spreads first through the right atrium and then into the left atrium. Thus the sinus node functions as the normal *pacemaker* of the heart.

The first phase of cardiac muscle activation is electrical stimulation of the right and left atria. This in turn signals the atria to contract and pump blood simultaneously through the tricuspid and mitral valves into the right and left ventricles. The electrical stimulus then spreads to specialized conduction tissues in the *atrioventricular* (AV) *junc-tion,* which includes the *AV node* and *bundle of His,* and then into the *left* and *right bundle branches,* which transmit the stimulus to the ventricular muscle cells.

The AV junction, which acts as a sort of electri-cal "bridge" connecting the atria and ventricles, is located at the base of the interatrial septum and extends into the interventricular septum (see Fig. 1.1). The upper (proximal) part of the AV junction is the AV node. (In some texts the terms *AV node* and *AV junction* are used synonymously.) The lower (distal) part of the AV junction is called the *bundle of His* after the physiologist who de-scribed it. The bundle of His then divides into two main branches: the right bundle branch, which distributes the stimulus to the right ventricle, and the left bundle branch,* which distributes the stimulus to the left ventricle (see Fig. 1.1).

The electrical stimulus spreads simultaneously down the left and right bundle branches into

---

*As discussed in Chapter 3, the ECG actually records the *differences* in potential between these electrodes.

*The left bundle branch has two major subdivisions called *fascicles.* (These small bundles are discussed in Chapter 7 along with the *hemiblocks.*)

Conduction System of the Heart

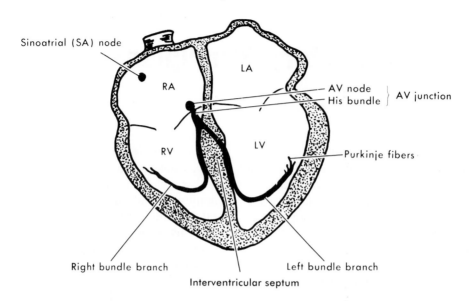

Fig. 1.1 Normally the cardiac stimulus is generated in the *sinoatrial (SA) node*, which is located in the *right atrium (RA)*. The stimulus then spreads through the *RA* and *left atrium (LA)*. Next, it spreads through the *atrioventricular (AV) node* and the *bundle of His*, which comprise the *AV junction*. The stimulus then passes into the *left* and *right ventricles (LV* and *RV)* by way of the *left* and *right bundle branches*, which are continuations of the bundle of His. Finally, the cardiac stimulus spreads to the ventricular muscle cells through the *Purkinje fibers.*

the *ventricular myocardium* (ventricular muscle) by way of specialized conducting cells called *Purkinje fibers*. These fibers are located in the ventricular myocardium.

Under normal circumstances, when the sinus node is pacing the heart (normal sinus rhythm), the AV junction appears to serve primarily as a shuttle, directing the electrical stimulus into the ventricles. However, under some circumstances the AV junction can also act as an independent pacemaker of the heart. For example, if the sinus node fails to function properly, the AV junction can act as an *escape* pacemaker. In such cases an AV junctional rhythm (and *not* sinus rhythm) is present. This produces a distinct ECG pattern (see Chapter 12).

Just as the spread of electrical stimuli through the atria leads to atrial contraction, so the spread of stimuli through the ventricles leads to ventricular contraction, with pumping of blood to the lungs and into the general circulation.

CARDIAC CONDUCTIVITY AND AUTOMATICITY

The speed with which electrical impulses are conducted through different parts of the heart varies. For example, conduction is *slowest* through the AV node and *fastest* through the Purkinje fibers. The relatively slow conduction speed through the AV node is of functional importance because it allows the ventricles time to fill with blood before the signal for cardiac contraction arrives.

In addition to *conductivity,* a major electrical feature of the heart is *automaticity.* Automaticity refers to the capacity of certain cardiac cells to function as pacemakers by spontaneously generating electrical impulses that spread throughout the heart. As mentioned earlier, the sinus node normally is the primary pacemaker of the heart because of its inherent automaticity. Under special conditions, however, other cells outside the sinus node (in the atria, AV junction, or ventricles) can also act as independent pacemakers. For example, if the automaticity of the sinus node is depressed, the AV junction can act as a secondary or escape pacemaker.

The term *sick sinus syndrome* is used clinically to describe patients who have severe depression of sinus node function (see Chapter 18). These patients may experience light-headedness or even syncope (fainting) because of excessive *bradycardia* (slow heartbeat). (Sick sinus syndrome and other causes of bradycardia are discussed in Part 2 in the section on cardiac arrhythmias.)

In other conditions the automaticity of pacemakers outside the sinus node may be abnormally increased, and these *ectopic* (nonsinus) pacemakers may compete with the sinus node for control of the heartbeat. A rapid run of ectopic beats results in an abnormal *tachycardia*. (Ectopy is also discussed in detail in Part 2.)

If you understand the normal physiologic stimulation of the heart, you have the basis for understanding the abnormalities of heart rhythm and conduction that produce distinctive ECG patterns. For example, failure of the sinus node to stimulate the heart properly can result in various rhythm disturbances associated with sick sinus syndrome. Blockage of the spread of stimuli through the AV junction can produce various degrees of AV heart block (see Chapter 15). Disease of the bundle branches can produce left or right bundle branch block (see Chapter 7). Finally, any disease process that involves the ventricular muscle itself (e.g., destruction of the heart muscle by myocardial infarction) can produce marked changes in the normal ECG patterns.

The first part of this book is devoted to explaining the basis of the normal ECG and then examining the major conditions that cause abnormal P, QRS, and T patterns.* The second part of the book is devoted to describing various abnormal rhythms *(arrhythmias)* and AV conduction disturbances. The third part of the book is a collection of "unknowns" for self-assessment. In addition, review questions are included at the end of each chapter. Selected publications are cited in the Bibliography.

---

*P, QRS, and T are defined in Chapter 2.

Review

An *electrocardiogram* (*ECG* or *EKG*) records the electrical voltages (potentials) produced in the heart. It does this by means of metal *electrodes* (connected to an electrocardiograph) placed on the patient's chest wall and extremities. The potentials recorded on the ECG are produced by the atrial and ventricular muscle fibers themselves.

Normally, the cardiac stimulus starts in pacemaker cells of the *sinus node,* also called the *sinoatrial (SA) node,* located high in the right atrium near the superior vena cava. From there the stimulus spreads downward and to the left, through the right and left atria, and reaches the *atrioventricular (AV) node,* located near the top of the interventricular septum (see Fig. 1.1). After a delay, the stimulus spreads through the *AV junction* (*AV node* and *bundle of His*). The bundle of His then subdivides into *right* and *left bundle branches.* The right bundle branch runs down the interventricular septum and into the right ventricle. From there the small *Purkinje fibers* rapidly distribute the stimulus outward into the main muscle mass of the right ventricle. Simultaneously, the left main bundle branch carries the stimulus down the interventricular septum to the muscle mass of the left ventricle, also by way of the Purkinje fibers.

This repetitive sequence of stimulation of the heart is the normal basic process. Disturbances in this process may produce abnormalities of heart rhythm, termed *cardiac arrhythmias.*

Questions

1. Label the major parts of the cardiac conduction system shown in this diagram; then trace the spread of the normal cardiac stimulus from the atria to the ventricles.

2. What is an electrocardiogram?

Basic ECG Waves

Depolarization and Repolarization

In Chapter 1 the general term electrical *stimulation* was applied to the spread of electrical stimuli through the atria and ventricles. The technical term for this cardiac electrical stimulation is *depolarization.* The return of heart muscle cells to their resting state following stimulation (depolarization) is called *repolarization.* These terms are derived from the fact that normal "resting" myocardial cells (atrial and ventricular cells) are polarized; that is, they carry electrical charges on their surface. Fig. 2.1, *A,* shows the resting polarized state of a normal atrial or ventricular heart muscle cell. Notice that the outside of the resting cell is positive and the inside is negative (about −90 mV).*

When a heart muscle cell is stimulated, it depolarizes. As a result the outside of the cell, in the area where the stimulation has occurred, becomes negative and the inside of the cell becomes positive. This produces a difference in electrical voltage on the outside surface of the cell between the stimulated depolarized area and the unstimulated polarized area (Fig. 2.1, *B*). Consequently, a small electrical current is formed that spreads along the length of the cell as stimulation and depolarization occur until the entire cell is depolarized (Fig. 2.1, *C*). The path of depolarization can be represented by an arrow, as shown in Fig. 2.1, *B.* For

individual myocardial cells (fibers), depolarization and repolarization proceed in the same direction. However, for the entire myocardium, depolarization proceeds from innermost layer (endocardium) to outermost layer (epicardium), whereas repolarization proceeds in the opposite direction. The mechanism of this difference is not fully understood.

The depolarizing electrical current is recorded by the ECG as a *P wave* (when the atria are stimulated and depolarize) and as a *QRS complex* (when the ventricles are stimulated and depolarize).

After a time the fully stimulated and depolarized cell begins to return to the resting state. This is known as *repolarization.* A small area on the outside of the cell becomes positive again (Fig. 2.1, *D*), and the repolarization spreads along the length of the cell until the entire cell is once again fully repolarized. Ventricular repolarization is recorded by the ECG as the *ST segment, T wave,* and *U wave.* (Atrial repolarization is usually obscured by ventricular potentials.)

The ECG records the electrical activity of a large mass of atrial and ventricular cells, not that of just a single cell. Because cardiac depolarization and repolarization normally occur in a synchronized fashion, the ECG is able to record these electrical currents as specific waves (P wave, QRS complex, ST segment, T wave, and U wave).

In summary, regardless of whether the ECG is normal or abnormal, it records just two basic events: (1) depolarization, the spread of a stimulus through the heart muscle, and (2) repolarization, the return of the stimulated heart muscle to the resting state.

---

*Membrane polarization is due to differences in the concentration of ions inside and outside the cell. See the Bibliography for references that present the electrophysiology of the *resting membrane potential* and *cellular depolarization* and *repolarization* (the action potential).

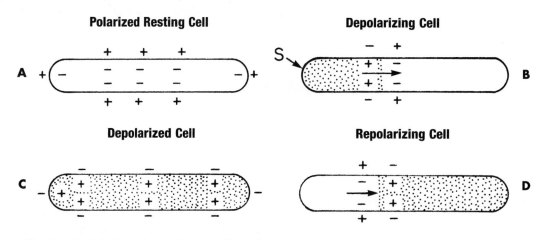

Fig. 2.1 Depolarization and repolarization. **A,** The resting heart muscle cell is polarized; that is, it carries an electrical charge, with the outside of the cell positively charged and the inside negatively charged. **B,** When the cell is stimulated *(S),* it begins to depolarize (stippled area). **C,** The fully depolarized cell is positively charged on the inside and negatively charged on the outside. **D,** Repolarization occurs when the stimulated cell returns to the resting state. The direction of depolarization and repolarization is represented by arrows. Depolarization (stimulation) of the atria produces the P wave on the ECG, whereas depolarization of the ventricles produces the QRS complex. Repolarization of the ventricles produces the ST-T complex.

Basic ECG Complexes: P, QRS, ST, T, and U Waves

The spread of stimuli through the atria and ventricles followed by the return of stimulated atrial and ventricular muscle to the resting state produces the electrical currents recorded on the ECG. Furthermore, each phase of cardiac electrical activity produces a specific wave or complex (Fig. 2.2). The basic ECG waves are labeled alphabetically and begin with the P wave:

- P wave—atrial depolarization (stimulation)
- QRS complex—ventricular depolarization (stimulation)
- ST segment, T wave, and U wave—ventricular repolarization (recovery)

The P wave represents the spread of a stimulus through the atria (atrial depolarization). The QRS complex represents stimulus spread through the ventricles (ventricular depolarization). The ST segment and T wave represent the return of stimulated ventricular muscle to the resting state (ventricular repolarization). The U wave is a small deflection sometimes seen just after the T wave. It represents the final phase of ventricular repolarization although its exact mechanism is not known.

Basic ECG Complexes

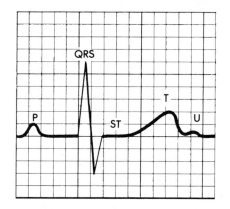

Fig. 2.2 The P wave represents atrial depolarization. The PR interval is the time from initial stimulation of the atria to initial stimulation of the ventricles. The QRS represents ventricular depolarization. The ST segment, T wave, and U wave are produced by ventricular repolarization.

You are probably wondering why no wave or complex represents the return of stimulated atria to their resting state. The answer is that the atrial ST segment (STa) and atrial T wave (Ta) are generally not observed on the normal ECG because of

Cardiac Electrical Cycle

Fig. 2.3 The basic cardiac cycle (P-QRS-T) repeats itself again and again.

their low amplitudes. (An important exception is described in Chapter 10 in the discussion of pericarditis.) Similarly, the routine ECG is not sensitive enough to record any electrical activity during the spread of stimuli through the atrioventricular (AV) junction (AV node and bundle of His). The spread of electrical stimuli through the AV junction occurs between the beginning of the P wave and the beginning of the QRS complex. This interval, known as the *PR interval,* is a measure of the time it takes for a stimulus to spread through the atria and pass through the AV junction.

In summary, the P-QRS-T sequence represents the repetitive cycle of the electrical activity in the heart, beginning with the spread of a stimulus through the atria (P wave) and ending with the return of stimulated ventricular muscle to its resting state (ST-T sequence). As shown in Fig. 2.3, this cardiac cycle repeats itself again and again.

ECG Paper

The P-QRS-T sequence is recorded on special ECG graph paper that is divided into gridlike boxes (Figs. 2.3 and 2.4). Each of the small boxes is 1 millimeter square (1 mm²). The paper usually moves at a speed of 25 mm/sec. Therefore horizontally, each unit represents 0.04 second (25 mm/sec × 0.04 sec = 1 mm). Notice that the lines between every five boxes are heavier, so that each 5-mm

unit horizontally corresponds to 0.2 second (5 × 0.04 = 0.2). The ECG can therefore be regarded as a moving graph that horizontally corresponds to time, with 0.04- and 0.2-second divisions.

Vertically the ECG graph measures the voltages, or amplitudes, of the ECG waves or deflections. The exact voltages can be measured because the electrocardiograph is standardized (calibrated) so that a 1-mV signal produces a deflection of 10-mm amplitude (1 mV = 10 mm). In most electrocardiographs the standardization can also be set at one-half or two-times normal sensitivity.

Basic ECG Measurements and Some Normal Values

STANDARDIZATION MARK

The electrocardiograph must be properly calibrated so that a 1-mV signal produces a 10-mm deflection. The unit may have a special standardization button that produces a 1-mV wave. As shown in Fig. 2.5, the standardization mark (St) produced when the machine is correctly calibrated is a square wave 10 mm tall. If the machine is not standardized correctly, the 1-mV signal produces a deflection either more or less than 10 mm and the amplitudes of the P, QRS, and T deflections are larger or smaller than they should be. The standardization deflection is also important because standardization can be varied in most electrocardiographs (see Fig. 2.5).

When very large deflections are present (as occurs, for example, in some patients who have an electronic pacemaker that produces very large spikes or who have high QRS voltage caused by hypertrophy), it may be advisable to take the ECG at one-half standardization to get the entire tracing on the paper. If the ECG complexes are very small, it may be advisable to double the standardization (e.g., to study a small Q wave more thoroughly). The standardization need be set only once on an ECG—just before the first lead is recorded.*

---

*Some electronic electrocardiographs do not display the calibration pulse. Instead, they print the paper speed and standardization at the bottom of the ECG paper (25 mm/sec, 10 mm/mV).

ECG Graph Paper

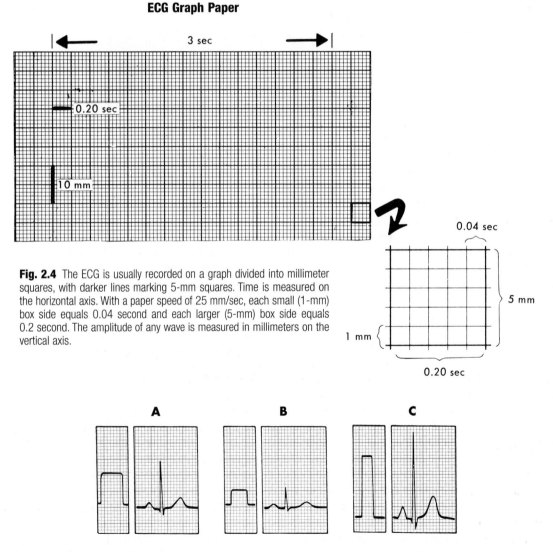

Fig. 2.4 The ECG is usually recorded on a graph divided into millimeter squares, with darker lines marking 5-mm squares. Time is measured on the horizontal axis. With a paper speed of 25 mm/sec, each small (1-mm) box side equals 0.04 second and each larger (5-mm) box side equals 0.2 second. The amplitude of any wave is measured in millimeters on the vertical axis.

Fig. 2.5 Before taking an ECG, the operator must check to see that the machine is properly calibrated, so that the 1-mV standardization mark is 10 mm tall. **A,** Electrocardiograph set at normal standardization. **B,** One-half standardization. **C,** Two times normal standardization.

Because the ECG is calibrated, any part of the P, QRS, and T deflections can be described in two ways; that is, both the amplitude (voltage) and the width (duration) of deflection can be measured. Thus it is possible to measure the amplitude and width of the P wave, the amplitude and width of the QRS complex, the amplitude of the ST segment deviation (if present), and the amplitude of the T wave. For clinical purposes, if the standardization is set at 1 mV = 10 mm, the height of a wave is usually recorded in millimeters, not millivolts. In Fig. 2.3, for example, the

P wave is 1 mm in amplitude, the QRS complex is 8 mm, and the T wave is about 3.5 mm.

A wave or deflection is also described as positive or negative. By convention, an *upward* deflection or wave is called *positive*. A *downward* deflection or wave is called *negative*. A deflection or wave that rests on the baseline is said to be *isoelectric*. A deflection that is partly positive and partly negative is call *biphasic*. For example, in Fig. 2.6 the P wave is positive, the QRS complex is biphasic (initially positive, then negative), the ST segment is isoelectric (flat on the baseline), and the T wave is negative.

The P, QRS, ST, T, and U waves are examined in a general way in this chapter. The measurements of heart rate, PR interval, QRS width, and QT interval are considered in detail, along with their normal values.

P WAVE

The P wave, which represents atrial depolarization, is a small positive (or negative) deflection before the QRS complex. (The normal values for P wave amplitude and width are described in Chapter 6.)

PR INTERVAL

The PR interval is measured from the beginning of the P wave to the beginning of the QRS complex (Fig. 2.7). The PR interval may vary slightly in different leads, and the shortest PR interval should

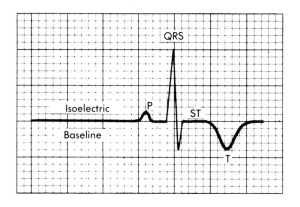

Fig. 2.6 The P wave is positive (upward), and the T wave is negative (downward). The QRS complex is biphasic (partly positive, partly negative), and the ST segment is isoelectric (neither positive nor negative).

Fig. 2.7 Measurement of the PR interval (see text).

be noted. The PR interval represents the time it takes for the stimulus to spread through the atria and pass through the AV junction. (This physiologic delay allows the ventricles to fill fully with blood before ventricular depolarization occurs.) *In adults the normal PR interval is between 0.12 and 0.2 second (three to five small box sides).* When conduction through the AV junction is impaired, the PR interval may become prolonged. Prolongation of the PR interval above 0.2 second is called *first-degree heart block* (see Chapter 15).

QRS NOMENCLATURE

One of the most confusing aspects of electrocardiography for the beginning student is the nomenclature of the QRS complex. As noted previously, the QRS complex represents the spread of a stimulus through the ventricles. However, not every QRS complex contains a Q wave, an R wave, and an S wave—hence the confusion. The bothersome but unavoidable nomenclature becomes understandable if you remember several

basic features of the QRS complex (Fig. 2.8): When the initial deflection of the QRS complex is negative (below the baseline), it is called a *Q wave.* The first positive deflection in the QRS complex is called an *R wave.* A negative deflection following the R wave is called an *S wave.* Thus the following QRS complex contains a Q wave, an R wave, and an S wave:

In contrast, the following complex does not contain three waves:

If, as shown above, the entire QRS complex is positive, it is simply called an *R wave.* However, if

How to Name the QRS Complex

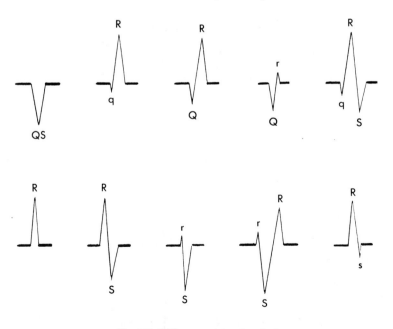

Fig. 2.8 QRS nomenclature (see text).

the entire complex is negative, it is termed a *QS wave* (not just a Q wave as you might expect).

Occasionally the QRS complex contains more than two or three deflections. In such cases the extra waves are called *R'* (R prime) *waves* if they are positive and *S'* (S prime) *waves* if they are negative.

Fig. 2.8 shows the various possible QRS complexes and the nomenclature of the respective waves. Notice that capital letters (QRS) are used to designate waves of relatively large amplitude and small letters (qrs) label relatively small waves (see Fig. 2.8).

The QRS nomenclature is confusing at first, but it allows you to describe any QRS complex over the phone and to evoke in the mind of the trained listener an exact mental picture of the complex named. For example, in describing an ECG you might say that lead V_1 showed an rS complex ("small r, capital S"):

You might also describe a QS ("capital Q, capital S") in lead aV_F:

QRS WIDTH (INTERVAL)

The QRS width, or interval, represents the time required for a stimulus to spread through the ventricles (ventricular depolarization) and is nor-mally 0.1 second or less (Fig. 2.9). If the spread of a stimulus through the ventricles is slowed, for example by a block in one of the bundle branches, the QRS width is prolonged. (The full differential diagnosis of a wide QRS complex is discussed in Chapters 10 and 22.)

ST SEGMENT

The ST segment is that portion of the ECG cycle from the end of the QRS complex to the beginning of the T wave (Fig. 2.10). It represents the beginning of ventricular repolarization. The normal ST segment is usually *isoelectric* (i.e., flat on the baseline, neither positive nor negative), but it may be slightly elevated or depressed normally (usually by less than 1 mm). Some pathologic conditions such as myocardial infarction (MI) produce characteristic abnormal deviations of the ST segment. The very beginning of the ST segment (actually the junction between the end of the QRS complex and the beginning of the ST segment) is sometimes called the *J point*. Fig. 2.10 shows the J point and the normal shapes of the ST segment. Fig. 2.11 compares a normal isoelectric ST segment with abnormal ST segment elevation and depression.

T WAVE

The T wave represents part of ventricular repolarization. A normal T wave has an asymmetric shape; that is, its peak is closer to the end of the wave than to the beginning (see Fig. 2.10). When the T wave is positive, it normally rises slowly and

QRS Interval

Fig. 2.9 Measurement of the QRS width (interval) (see text).

J Point, ST Segment, and T Wave

Fig. 2.10 Characteristics of the normal ST segment and T wave. The junction *(J)* is the beginning of the ST segment.

then abruptly returns to the baseline.* When it is negative, it descends slowly and abruptly rises to the baseline. The *asymmetry* of the normal T wave contrasts with the symmetry of T waves in certain abnormal conditions such as MI (see Chapters 8 and 9) and a high serum potassium level (see Chapter 10).

QT INTERVAL

The QT interval is measured from the beginning of the QRS complex to the end of the T wave (Fig. 2.12). It primarily represents the return of stimulated ventricles to their resting state (ventricular repolarization). The normal values

---

*The exact point at which the ST segment ends and the T wave begins is arbitrary and sometimes impossible to define.

for the QT interval depend on the heart rate. As the heart rate increases (RR interval* shortens), the QT normally shortens; as the heart rate decreases (RR interval lengthens), the QT interval lengthens.

The QT interval should be measured in the ECG leads (see Chapter 3) that show the largest-amplitude T waves. You should measure several intervals and use the average value. When the QT interval is long, it is often difficult to measure because the end of the T wave may merge imperceptibly with the U wave. As a result, you may be measuring the QU interval rather than the QT interval.

Table 2.1 shows the upper normal limits for the QT interval with different heart rates. Unfortunately, there is no simple rule for calculating the normal limits of the QT interval.

Because of this problem, another index of the QT has been devised. It is the *rate-corrected* QT or

---

*The interval between QRS complexes is termed the *RR interval*.

ST Segments

Fig. 2.11 ST segments. **A,** Normal. **B,** Abnormal elevation. **C,** Abnormal depression.

Table 2.1	QT Interval: Upper Limits of Normal	
Measured RR interval (sec)	**Heart rate (per min)**	**QT interval upper normal limits (sec)**
1.50	40	0.50
1.20	50	0.45
1.00	60	0.42
0.86	70	0.40
0.80	75	0.38
0.75	80	0.37
0.67	90	0.35
0.60	100	0.34
0.50	120	0.31
0.40	150	0.25

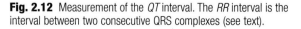

Fig. 2.12 Measurement of the *QT* interval. The *RR* interval is the interval between two consecutive QRS complexes (see text).

QT$_c$. The rate-corrected QT is obtained by dividing the actual QT by the square root of the RR interval (both measured in seconds):

$$QT_c = \frac{QT}{\sqrt{RR}}$$

Normally the QT$_c$ is less than or equal to 0.44 second.

A number of factors can abnormally prolong the QT interval (Fig. 2.13). For example, this interval can be prolonged by certain drugs (e.g., quinidine, procainamide, disopyramide, sotalol, amiodarone) and by electrolyte disturbances (a low serum potassium or low serum calcium level). Hypothermia also prolongs the QT interval by slowing the repolarization of myocardial cells. The QT interval may be prolonged with myocardial ischemia and infarction and with subarachnoid hemorrhage. QT prolongation may predispose patients to potentially lethal ventricular arrhythmias. (See the discussion of torsade de pointes in Chapters 14 and 22.)

Fig. 2.13 Abnormal QT interval prolongation in a patient taking quinidine. The QT interval (0.6 second) is markedly prolonged for the heart rate (65 beats/min) (see Table 2.1). The rate-corrected QT interval (normally 0.44 second or less) is also prolonged (0.63 second).* Prolonged polarization may predispose patients to develop torsade de pointes, a life-threatening ventricular arrhythmia (see Chapter 14).

---

*In Fig. 2.13, find the QT$_c$.

$$\frac{QT}{\sqrt{RR}} = \frac{0.60}{\sqrt{0.92}} = 0.63$$

The QT interval may also be shortened, for example, by digitalis in therapeutic doses or by hypercalcemia. Because the lower limits of normal for the QT interval have not been well defined, only the upper limits are given in Table 2.1.

U WAVE

The U wave is a small, rounded deflection sometimes seen after the T wave (see Fig. 2.2). As noted previously, its exact significance is not known. Functionally, U waves represent the last phase of ventricular repolarization. Prominent U waves are characteristic of hypokalemia (see Chapter 10). Very prominent U waves may also be seen in other settings, for example, in patients taking drugs such as quinidine or one of the phenothiazines or sometimes after patients have had a cerebrovascular accident. The appearance of very prominent U waves in such settings, with or without actual QT prolongation, may also predispose patients to ventricular arrhythmias (see Chapter 14).

Normally the direction of the U wave is the same as that of the T wave. Negative U waves sometimes appear with positive T waves. This abnormal finding has been noted in left ventricular hypertrophy and myocardial ischemia.

CALCULATION OF HEART RATE

Two simple methods can be used to measure the heart rate (number of heartbeats per minute) from the ECG:

1. The easier way, when the heart rate is regular, is to count the number of large (0.2-sec) boxes between two successive QRS complexes and divide a constant (300) by this. (The number of large time boxes is divided into 300 because $300 \times 0.2 = 60$ and the heart rate is being calculated in beats per minute or 60 seconds.)

   For example, in Fig. 2.14 the heart rate is 75 beats/min, since four large time boxes are counted between successive R waves ($300 \div 4 = 75$). Similarly, if two large time boxes are counted between successive R waves, the heart rate is 150 beats/min. With five intervening large time boxes, the heart rate is 60 beats/min.

When the heart rate must be measured very accurately from the ECG, you can modify the approach as follows: Count the number of small (0.04 sec) boxes between successive R waves and divide a constant (1500) by this number. In Fig. 2.4, 20 small time boxes are counted between QRS complexes. Therefore the heart rate is 1500 ÷ 20 = 75 beats/min. (The constant 1500 is used because 1500 × 0.04 = 60 and the heart rate is being calculated in beats per 60 seconds.)

2. If the heart rate is irregular, the first method will not be accurate because the intervals between QRS complexes vary from beat to beat. In such cases you can determine an average rate simply

What Is the Heart Rate?

Fig. 2.14 Heart rate (beats per minute) can be measured by counting the number of large (0.2 second) time boxes between two successive QRS complexes and dividing 300 by this number. In this example the heart rate is calculated as 300 ÷ 4 = 75 beats/min.

by counting the number of cardiac *cycles* every 6 seconds and multiplying this number by 10 (Fig. 2.15). (A cardiac cycle is the interval between two successive R waves.) Counting the number of cardiac cycles every 6 seconds can be easily done because the top of the ECG paper, as shown in Fig. 2.14, is generally scored with vertical marks every 3 seconds.*

By definition, a heart rate exceeding 100 beats/min is termed *tachycardia,* and a heart rate slower than 60 beats/min is called *bradycardia.* (In Greek, *tachys* means "swift," whereas *bradys* means "slow.") Thus during exercise you probably develop a sinus tachycardia, but during sleep or relaxation your pulse rate may drop into the 50s or even lower, indicating a sinus bradycardia.

The ECG as a Combination of Atrial and Ventricular Parts

The ECG really consists of two separate but normally related parts: an atrial ECG, represented by the P wave, and a ventricular ECG, repre-

*If 3-second marks are not present, you can simply count the number of QRS cycles in any 15-cm interval and multiply this number by 10. On the ECG graph, 1 second = 25 mm = 2.5 cm; therefore 15 cm 5 6 seconds of data.

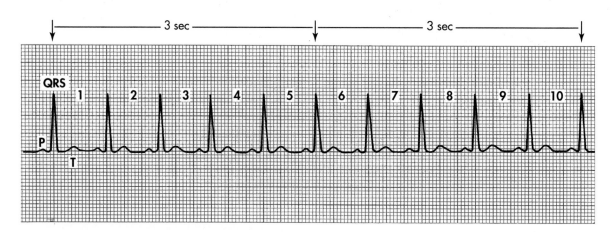

Fig. 2.15 Measurement of heart rate (beats per minute) by counting the number of cardiac cycles in a 6-second interval and multiplying this number by 10. In this example, 10 cardiac cycles occur in 6 seconds. Therefore the heart rate is 10 × 10 = 100 beats/min. The arrows point to 3-second markers.

sented by the QRS-T sequence. With completely normal rhythm, when the sinus node is pacing the heart, the P wave (atrial stimulation or depolarization) always precedes the QRS complex (ventricular stimulation or depolarization) because the atria are electrically stimulated first. Therefore the P-QRS-T cycle is usually considered as a unit. However, in some abnormal conditions the atria and the ventricles can be stimulated by separate pacemakers. For example, suppose that the AV junction is diseased and stimuli cannot pass from the atria to the ventricles. In this situation a new (subsidiary) pacemaker located below the level of the block in the AV junction may take over the task of pacing the ventricles while the sinus node continues to pace the atria. In this case, stimulation of the atria is independent of stimulation of the ventricles, and the P waves and QRS complexes have no relation to each other. This type of arrhythmia is called *complete heart block* and is described in detail in Chapter 15 (Fig. 15.5 shows an example of this abnormal condition in which the atrial and ventricular ECGs are independent of each other.)

The ECG in Perspective

Up to this point only the basic components of the ECG have been considered. Several general items need to be emphasized before actual ECG patterns are discussed.

1. The ECG is a recording of cardiac *electrical* activity. It does not directly measure the *mechanical* function of the heart (i.e., how well the heart is contracting and performing as a pump). Thus a patient with acute pulmonary edema may have a normal ECG. Conversely, a patient with a grossly abnormal ECG may have normal cardiac function.

2. The ECG does not directly depict abnormalities in cardiac structure such as ventricular septal defects and abnormalities of the heart valves. It only records the electrical changes produced by structural defects. However, in some patients a specific structural diagnosis such as mitral stenosis, pulmonary embolism, or MI can be inferred from the ECG because typical electrical abnormalities may develop in such patients.

3. The ECG does not record *all* the heart's electrical activity. The electrodes placed on the surface of the body record only the currents that are transmitted to the area of electrode placement. Therefore there are actually "silent" electrical areas of the heart. For example, the ECG is not sensitive enough to record depolarization of pacemaker cells in the sinus node occurring just before the P wave. As noted earlier, repolarization of the atria generally is not recorded by the conventional electrocardiograph. (For an important exception, see the discussion of pericarditis in Chapter 10.) Also, the spread of stimuli through the AV junction is not detected by the conventional ECG. The electrical activity of the AV junction can be recorded using a special apparatus and a special electrode placed in the heart *(His bundle electrogram)*. In addition, the ECG records the summation of electrical potentials produced by innumerable cardiac muscle cells. Therefore the presence of a normal ECG does not necessarily mean that all these heart muscle cells are being depolarized and repolarized in a normal way.

For these reasons the ECG must be regarded as any other laboratory test, with proper consideration for both its uses and its limitations (see Chapter 19).

The 12 ECG leads are described in Chapter 3. Normal and abnormal ECG patterns are discussed in subsequent chapters.

Review

The ECG, whether normal or abnormal, records two basic physiologic processes: *depolarization* and *repolarization:*

1. Depolarization (the spread of stimulus through the heart muscle) produces the P wave from the atria and the QRS complex from the ventricles.
2. Repolarization (the return of stimulated muscle to the resting state) produces the atrial ST segment and T wave (which are ordinarily not seen on the ECG) and the ventricular ST segment, T wave, and U wave.

ECGs are recorded on special paper that is divided into gridlike boxes. Each small box is 1 mm². Each millimeter horizontally represents 0.04 second. Each 0.2 second is denoted by a heavier vertical line. ECG deflections are usually standardized so that a 1-mV signal produces a 10-mm deflection. Therefore each millimeter vertically represents 0.1 mV. Each 5-mm interval is denoted by a heavier horizontal line.

Four basic intervals are measured on the ECG:

1. The *heart rate* (based on RR intervals) can be calculated in two ways:
   a. Method 1: Count the number of large (0.2-second) time boxes between two successive R waves, and divide the constant 300 by this number (see Fig. 2.14). If you want a more accurate measurement of the rate, divide the constant 1500 by the number of small (0.04-second) time boxes between two successive R waves.
   b. Method 2: Count the number of cardiac cycles that occur every 6 seconds, and multiply this number by 10. A vertical mark may be present on the top of the ECG paper every 3 seconds. A *cardiac cycle* is the interval between two successive QRS complexes.
2. The *PR interval* is measured from the beginning of the P wave to the beginning of the QRS complex. The normal PR interval varies from 0.12 to 0.2 second.
3. The *QRS interval* is normally 0.1 second or less in width.
4. The *QT interval* is measured from the beginning of the QRS complex to the end of the T wave. It varies with the heart rate, becoming shorter as the heart rate increases.

These four intervals can be considered the "vital signs" of the ECG because they give essential information about the electrical stability (or instability) of the heart.

Questions

1. Calculate the heart rate in each of the following examples:

2. Name the major abnormality in each example.

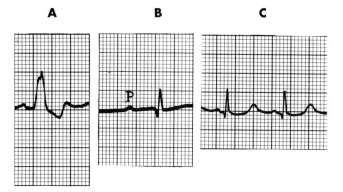

3. Slowing of conduction in the atrioventricular node is most likely to do which of the following?
   a. Prolong the PR interval
   b. Prolong the QRS interval
   c. Prolong the QT interval
   d. All of the above
4. A block in the left or right bundle branch is most likely to do which of the following?
   a. Prolong the PR interval
   b. Prolong the QRS interval
   c. Prolong the QT interval
   d. All of the above
5. Name the component waves of the QRS complexes shown below.

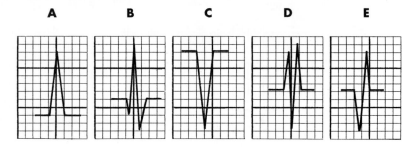

6. Name four factors that may prolong the QT interval.

ECG Leads

As discussed in Chapter 1, the heart produces electrical currents similar to the familiar dry cell battery. The strength or voltage of these currents and the way they are distributed throughout the body can be measured by a suitable recording instrument such as an electrocardiograph.

The body acts as a conductor of electricity. Therefore recording electrodes placed some distance from the heart, such as on the arms, legs, or chest wall, are able to detect the voltages of the cardiac currents conducted to these locations. *The usual way of recording these voltages from the heart is with the 12 standard ECG leads. The leads actually show the differences in voltage (potential) between electrodes placed on the surface of the body.*

Taking an ECG is like recording an event such as a baseball game with a video camera. Multiple camera angles are necessary to capture the event completely. One view is not enough. Similarly, multiple ECG leads must be recorded to describe the electrical activity of the heart adequately. Fig. 3.1 shows the ECG patterns that are obtained when electrodes are placed at various points on the chest. Notice that each lead presents a different pattern.

Fig. 3.2 is an ECG illustrating the 12 leads. The leads can be subdivided into two groups: the six *extremity (limb)* leads (shown in the left two columns) and the six *chest (precordial)* leads (shown in the right two columns).

The six extremity leads—I, II, III, aV_R, aV_L, and aV_F—record voltage differences by means of electrodes placed on the limbs. They can be further divided into two subgroups: the *bipolar* extremity leads (I, II, and III) and the *unipolar* extremity leads (aV_R, aV_L, and aV_F).

The six chest leads—V_1, V_2, V_3, V_4, V_5, and V_6—record voltage differences by means of electrodes placed at various positions on the chest wall.

The 12 ECG leads can also be viewed as 12 "channels." However, in contrast to television channels (which can be tuned to different events), the 12 ECG channels (leads) are all tuned to the *same* event (the P-QRS-T cycle), with each lead viewing the event from a different angle.

Extremity (Limb) Leads

BIPOLAR LEADS (I, II, AND III)

The extremity leads are recorded first. In connecting a patient to an electrocardiograph, first place metal electrodes on the arms and legs. The right leg electrode functions solely as an electrical ground, so you need concern yourself with it no further. As shown in Fig. 3.3, the arm electrodes are attached just above the wrist and the leg electrodes are attached above the ankles.

The electrical voltages of the heart are conducted through the torso to the extremities. Therefore an electrode placed on the right wrist detects electrical voltages equivalent to those recorded below the right shoulder. Similarly, the voltages detected at the left wrist or anywhere else on the left arm are equivalent to those recorded below the left shoulder. Finally, voltages detected by the left leg electrode are comparable to those at the left thigh or near the groin. In clinical practice the electrodes are attached to the wrists and ankles simply for convenience.*

---

*Obviously, if you are taking an ECG on an amputee or someone with a cast, you have to place the electrodes below or near the shoulders or groin, depending on the circumstance.

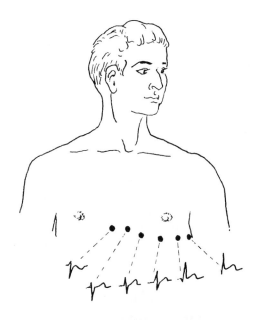

Fig. 3.1 Multiple chest leads give a three-dimensional view of cardiac electrical activity.

As mentioned, the extremity leads consist of bipolar (I, II, and III) and unipolar (aV_R, aV_L, and aV_F) leads. The bipolar leads are so named because they record the differences in electrical voltage between two extremities.

Lead I, for example, records the difference in voltage between the left arm (LA) and right arm (RA) electrodes:

$$\text{Lead I} = \text{LA} - \text{RA}$$

Lead II records the difference between the left leg (LL) and right arm (RA) electrodes:

$$\text{Lead II} = \text{LL} - \text{RA}$$

Lead III records the difference between the left leg (LL) and left arm (LA) electrodes:

$$\text{Lead III} = \text{LL} - \text{LA}$$

Consider what happens when you turn on the electrocardiograph to lead I. The LA electrode detects the electrical voltages of the heart that are transmitted to the left arm. The RA electrode detects the voltages transmitted to the

Fig. 3.2 A, Sample ECG showing the 12 standard leads. **B,** A lead II rhythm strip. What is the approximate heart rate? (Answer: 50 to 60 beats/min.)

right arm. Inside the electrocardiograph the RA voltages are subtracted from the LA voltages, and the difference appears at lead I. When lead II is recorded, a similar situation occurs between the voltages of LL and RA. When lead III is recorded, the same situation occurs between the voltages of LL and LA.

Leads I, II, and III can be represented schematically in terms of a triangle, called *Einthoven's triangle* after the Dutch physician who invented the electrocardiograph in the early 1900s. At first the ECG consisted only of recordings from leads I, II, and III. Einthoven's triangle (Fig. 3.4) shows the spatial orientation of the three bipolar extremity leads (I, II, and III). As you can see, lead I points horizontally. Its left pole (LA) is positive and its right pole (RA) is negative. Therefore lead I = LA − RA. Lead II points diagonally downward. Its lower pole (LL) is positive and its upper pole (RA) is negative. Therefore lead II = LL − RA. Lead III also points diagonally downward. Its lower pole (LL) is positive and its upper pole (LA) is negative. Therefore lead III = LL − LA.

Einthoven, of course, could have hooked the leads up differently. Yet because of the way he arranged them, the bipolar leads are related by the following simple equation:

$$\text{Lead I} + \text{Lead III} = \text{Lead II}$$

In other words, add the voltage in lead I to that in lead III and you get the voltage in lead II.* You can test this equation by looking at Fig. 3.2. Add the voltage of the R wave in lead I (+9 mm) to the voltage of the R wave in lead III (+4 mm) and you get +13 mm, the voltage of the R wave in lead II. You can do the same with the voltages of the P waves and T waves.

---

*This rule is only approximate. It is exact when the three bipolar extremity leads are recorded simultaneously, using a three-channel electrocardiograph, because the peaks of the R waves in the three leads do *not* occur simultaneously. The exact rule is as follows: the voltage at the peak of the R wave (or at any point) in lead II equals the sum of the voltages in leads I and III at points occurring simultaneously.

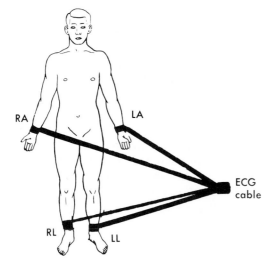

Fig. 3.3 Metal electrodes strapped on to take an ECG. The right leg *(RL)* electrode functions solely as a ground to prevent alternating-current interference. (*LA,* left arm; *RA,* right arm; *LL,* left leg.)

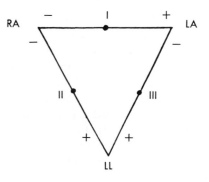

Fig. 3.4 Orientation of leads I, II, and III. Lead I records the difference in electrical potentials between the left arm and right arm. Lead II records it between the left leg and right arm. Lead III records it between the left leg and left arm.

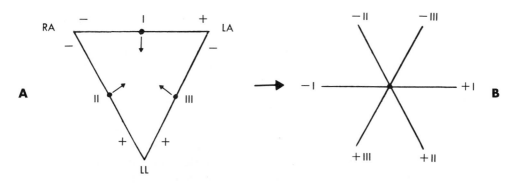

Fig. 3.5 A, Einthoven's triangle. **B,** The triangle is converted to a triaxial diagram by shifting leads I, II, and III so that they intersect at a common point.

It is a good practice to scan leads I, II, and III rapidly when you first look at a mounted ECG. If the R wave in lead II does not seem to be the sum of the R waves in leads I and II, this may be a clue that the leads have been recorded incorrectly or mounted improperly.

Einthoven's equation is simply the result of the way the bipolar leads are recorded; that is, the LA is positive in lead I and negative in lead III and thus cancels out when the two leads are added:

$$I = L\cancel{A} - RA$$
$$III = LL - L\cancel{A}$$
$$I + III = LL - RA = II$$

Thus in electrocardiography, one plus three equals two.

In summary, the first three leads (I, II, and III) are bipolar extremity leads, which historically were the first invented. These leads record the differences in electrical voltage between extremities.

In Fig. 3.5, Einthoven's triangle has been redrawn so that leads I, II, and III intersect at a common central point. This was done simply by sliding lead I downward, lead II rightward, and lead III leftward. The result is the *triaxial* diagram in Fig. 3.5, *B*. This diagram, a useful way of representing the three bipolar leads, is employed in Chapter 5.

UNIPOLAR EXTREMITY LEADS (aV$_R$, aV$_L$, AND aV$_F$)

Nine leads have been added to the original three bipolar extremity leads. In the 1930s, Dr. Frank N. Wilson and his colleagues at the University of Michigan invented the unipolar extremity leads and introduced the six unipolar chest leads, V$_1$ through V$_6$. A short time later, Dr. Emanuel Goldberger invented the three augmented unipolar extremity leads: aV$_R$, aV$_L$, and aV$_F$. The abbreviation *a* refers to *augmented; V* to *voltage; R, L,* and *F* to *right arm, left arm,* and *left foot* (leg) respectively. Today 12 leads are routinely employed.

A unipolar lead records the electrical voltages at one location relative to zero potential rather than relative to the voltages at another extremity, as in the case of the bipolar extremity leads.* The zero potential is obtained inside the electrocardiograph by joining the three extremity leads to a central terminal. Because the sum of the voltages of RA, LA, and LL equals zero, the central terminal has a zero voltage. The aV$_R$, aV$_L$, and aV$_F$ leads are derived in a slightly different way because the voltages recorded by the electrocardiograph have been augmented 50% over the actual voltages detected at each extremity. This augmentation is also done electronically inside the electrocardiograph.†

Just as Einthoven's triangle represents the spatial orientation of the three bipolar extremity leads, the diagram in Fig. 3.6 represents the spa-

---

*Although unipolar leads (like bipolar leads) are represented by axes with positive and negative poles, the term unipolar does not refer to these poles; rather it refers to the fact that unipolar leads record the voltage in one location relative to zero potential.

†Augmentation was developed to make the complexes more readable.

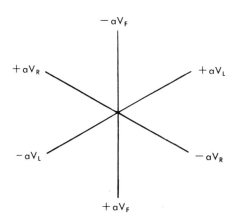

Fig. 3.6 Triaxial lead diagram showing the relationship of the three augmented unipolar leads (aV$_R$, aV$_L$, and aV$_F$). Notice that each lead is represented by an axis with a positive and negative pole. *Unipolar* means that the leads record the voltage in one location relative to zero potential.

tial orientation of the three unipolar extremity leads. Notice that each of the unipolar leads can also be represented by a line (axis) with a positive and negative pole. Because the diagram has three axes, it is also called a *triaxial* diagram.

As would be expected, the positive pole of lead aV$_R$, the right arm lead, points upward and to the patient's right arm. The positive pole of lead aV$_L$ points upward and to the patient's left arm. The positive pole of lead aV$_F$ points downward toward the patient's left foot.

Furthermore, just as leads I, II, and III are related by Einthoven's equation, so leads aV$_R$, aV$_L$, and aV$_F$ are related:

$$aV_R + aV_L + aV_F = 0$$

In other words, when the three unipolar extremity leads are recorded, their voltages should total zero. Thus the sum of the P wave voltages is zero, the sum of the QRS voltages is zero, and the sum of the T wave voltages is zero. Using Fig. 3.2, test this equation by adding the QRS voltages in the three unipolar extremity leads (aV$_R$, aV$_L$, and aV$_F$).

It is also a good practice to scan leads aV$_R$, aV$_L$, and aV$_F$ rapidly when you first look at a mounted ECG. If the sum of the waves in these three leads

does not equal zero, the leads may have been recorded incorrectly or mounted improperly.

The ECG leads, both bipolar and unipolar, have two major features, which have already been described. They have both a specific *orientation* and a specific *polarity.*

Thus the axis of lead I is oriented horizontally, and the axis of lead aV$_R$ points diagonally downward. The orientation of the bipolar leads is shown in Einthoven's triangle (see Fig. 3.5), and the orientation of the unipolar extremity leads is diagrammed in Fig. 3.6.

The second major feature of the ECG leads, their polarity, can be represented by a line (axis) with a positive and a negative pole. (The polarity and spatial orientation of the leads are discussed further in Chapters 4 and 5 when the normal ECG patterns seen in each lead are considered and the concept of electrical axis is explored.)

Do not be confused by the difference in meaning between ECG electrodes and ECG leads. An *electrode* is simply the metal plate used to detect the electrical currents of the heart in any location. An ECG *lead* shows the differences in voltage detected by electrodes. For example, lead I presents the differences in voltage detected by the left and right arm electrodes. Therefore a lead is a means of recording the differences in cardiac voltages obtained by different electrodes.

RELATIONSHIP BETWEEN UNIPOLAR AND BIPOLAR EXTREMITY LEADS

Einthoven's triangle in Fig. 3.4 shows the relationship of the three bipolar extremity leads (I, II, and III). Similarly, the triaxial diagram in Fig. 3.7 shows the relationship of the three unipolar extremity leads (aV$_R$, aV$_L$, and aV$_F$). For convenience, these two diagrams can be combined so that the axes of all six extremity leads intersect at a common point. The result is the *hexaxial* lead diagram shown in Fig. 3.7. The hexaxial diagram shows the spatial orientation of the six extremity leads (I, II, III, aV$_R$, aV$_L$, and aV$_F$).

The exact relationships among the three unipolar extremity leads and the three bipolar extremity leads can also be described mathematically. However, for present purposes, the

Derivation of Hexaxial Lead Diagram

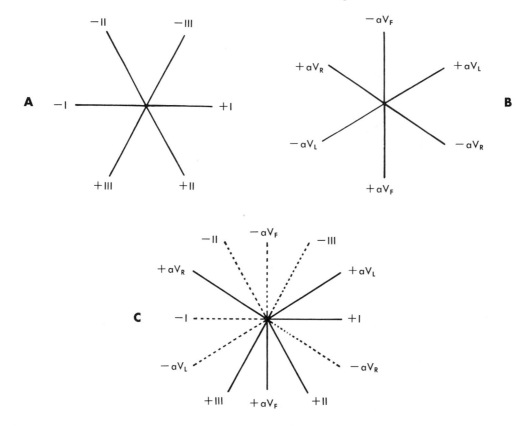

Fig. 3.7 A, Triaxial diagram of the bipolar leads (I, II, and III). **B,** Triaxial diagram of the unipolar leads (aV$_R$, aV$_L$, and aV$_F$). **C,** The two triaxial diagrams can be combined into a hexaxial diagram that shows the relationship of all six extremity leads. The negative pole of each lead is now indicated by a dashed line.

following simple guidelines allow you to get an overall impression of the similarities between these two sets of leads.

As you might expect by looking at the hexaxial diagram, the pattern in lead aV$_L$ usually resembles that in lead I. The positive poles of lead aV$_R$ and lead II, on the other hand, point in opposite directions. Therefore the P-QRS-T pattern recorded by lead aV$_R$ is generally the reverse of that recorded by lead II: For example, when lead II shows a qR pattern

lead aV$_R$ usually shows an rS pattern

Finally, the pattern shown by lead aV$_F$ usually but not always resembles that shown by lead III.

Chest (Precordial) Leads

The chest leads (V$_1$ to V$_6$) show the electrical currents of the heart as detected by electrodes placed at different positions on the chest wall. The precordial leads used today are also unipolar leads in that they measure the voltage in any one location

Chest Lead Placement

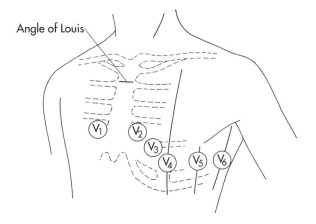

Fig. 3.8 Locations of the electrodes for the chest (precordial) leads.

Orientation of Chest Leads

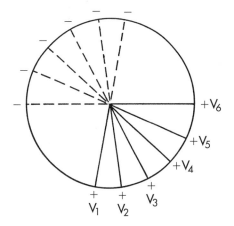

Fig. 3.9 The positive poles of the chest leads point anteriorly, and the negative poles *(dashed lines)* point posteriorly.

relative to zero potential (Box). The chest leads are recorded simply by means of electrodes (usually attached to suction cups to hold them in place on the chest) at six designated locations on the chest wall (Fig. 3.8).* Two points are worth mentioning here:

1. The fourth intercostal space can be located by placing your finger at the top of the sternum and moving it slowly downward. After you move your finger down about 1½ inches, you can feel a slight horizontal ridge. This is called the *angle of Louis,* which is located where the manubrium joins the body of the sternum (Fig. 3.8). The second intercostal space is just below and lateral to this point. Move down two more spaces. You are now in the fourth interspace and ready to place lead V_4.

2. Chest lead placement in females is complicated by breast tissue, which may result in misplacement of the chest leads. In taking ECGs on women, you must remember to place the electrode *under* the breast for leads

---

*Sometimes, in special circumstances (e.g., a patient with suspected congenital heart disease or right ventricular infarction), additional leads are placed on the right side of the chest. For example, lead V_{3R} is equivalent to lead V_3, but the electrode is placed to the right of the sternum.

Conventional Placement of ECG Chest Leads

Lead V_1 is recorded with the electrode in the fourth intercostal space just to the right of the sternum.
Lead V_2 is recorded with the electrode in the fourth intercostal space just to the left of the sternum.
Lead V_3 is recorded on a line midway between leads V_2 and V_4.
Lead V_4 is recorded in the midclavicular line in the fifth interspace.
Lead V_5 is recorded in the anterior axillary line at the same level as lead V_4.
Lead V_6 is recorded in the midaxillary line at the same level as lead V_4.

V_3 to V_6. If, as often happens, the electrode is placed *on* the breast, electrical voltages from higher interspaces are recorded. Also, never use the nipples to locate the position of any of the chest lead electrodes, even in men, because nipple location varies greatly in different persons.

The chest leads, like the six extremity leads, can be represented diagrammatically (Fig. 3.9). Like the other leads, each chest lead has a positive and negative pole. The positive pole of each chest lead points anteriorly, toward the front of the chest. The negative pole of each chest lead points posteriorly, toward the back (see the dashed lines in Fig. 3.9).

The 12-Lead ECG: Frontal and Horizontal Plane Leads

You may now be wondering why 12 leads are used in clinical electrocardiography. Why not 10 or 22 leads? The reason for exactly 12 leads is partly historical, a matter of the way the ECG has evolved over the years since Einthoven's original three bipolar extremity leads. There is nothing sacred about the electrocardiographer's dozen. In some situations, for example, additional leads are recorded by placing the chest electrode at different positions on the chest wall. Multiple leads are used for good reasons. The heart, after all, is a three-dimensional structure, and its electrical currents spread out in all directions across the body. Recall that the ECG leads were described as being like video cameras by which the electrical activity of the heart can be viewed from different locations. To a certain extent, the more points that are recorded, the more accurate the representation of the heart's electrical activity.

The importance of multiple leads is illustrated in the diagnosis of myocardial infarction (MI). An MI typically affects one localized portion of either the anterior or inferior portion of the left ventricle. The ECG changes produced by an anterior MI are usually best shown by the chest leads, which are close to and face the injured anterior surface of the heart. The changes seen with an inferior MI usually appear only in leads such as II, III, and aV$_F$, which face the injured inferior surface of the heart (see Chapters 8 and 9). The 12 leads therefore provide a three-dimensional view of the electrical activity of the heart.

Specifically, the six extremity leads (I, II, III, aV$_R$, aV$_L$, aV$_F$) record electrical voltages transmitted onto the *frontal* plane of the body (Fig. 3.10). (In contrast, the six precordial leads record voltages transmitted onto the *horizontal* plane.) For example, if you walk up to and face a large window, the window is parallel to the frontal plane of your body. Similarly, heart voltages directed upward and downward and to the right and left are recorded by the frontal plane leads.

The six chest leads (V$_1$ through V$_6$) record heart voltages transmitted onto the *horizontal* plane of the body (Fig. 3.11). The horizontal plane cuts your body into an upper and a lower half. Similarly, the chest leads record heart voltages directed anteriorly (front) and posteriorly (back), and to the right and left.

The 12 ECG leads are therefore divided into two sets: the six extremity leads (three unipolar and three bipolar), which record voltages on the frontal plane of the body, and the six chest (precordial) leads, which record voltages on the horizontal plane. Together these 12 leads provide a three-dimensional picture of atrial and ventricu-

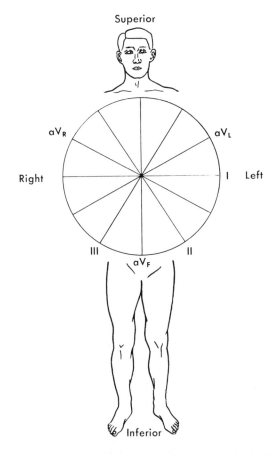

Fig. 3.10 Spatial relationships of the six extremity leads, which record electrical voltages transmitted onto the frontal plane of the body.

lar depolarization and repolarization. This multi-lead display is analogous to having 12 video cameras continuously recording cardiac electrical activity from different angles.

Cardiac Monitors and Monitor Leads

BEDSIDE CARDIAC MONITORS

Up to now, only the standard 12-lead ECG has been considered. However, it is not always necessary or feasible to record a full 12-lead ECG. For example, many patients require continuous monitoring for a prolonged period. In such cases, special cardiac monitors are used to give a continuous beat-to-beat record of cardiac activity from one monitor lead.

Fig. 3.12 is a rhythm strip recorded from a monitor lead obtained by means of three disk electrodes on the chest wall. As shown in Fig. 3.13, one electrode (the positive one) is usually pasted in the V_1 position. The other two are placed near the right and left shoulders. One serves as the negative electrode and the other as the ground.

When the location of the electrodes on the chest wall is varied, the resultant ECG patterns also vary. In addition, if the polarity of the electrodes changes (e.g., the negative electrode is con-

Horizontal Plane Leads

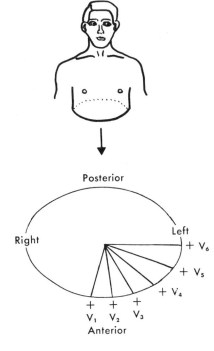

Fig. 3.11 Spatial relationships of the six chest leads, which record electrical voltages transmitted onto the horizontal plane.

Fig. 3.12 Rhythm strips from a cardiac monitor taken moments apart but showing exactly opposite patterns. This is because the polarity of the electrodes was reversed in the lower strip **(B).**

Electrode placement

Fig. 3.13 Monitor lead. A chest electrode *(+)* is placed at the lead V_1 position (between the fourth and fifth ribs on the right side of the sternum). The right shoulder acts as a negative *(−)* electrode. A ground electrode *(G)* is placed at the left shoulder. This lead is therefore a modified V_1.

nected to the V_1 position and the positive electrode to the right shoulder), the ECG shows a completely opposite pattern (see Fig. 3.12).

AMBULATORY MONITORS

The cardiac monitors just described are useful in patients confined to a bed or chair. Sometimes, however, heartbeat needs to be recorded in ambulatory patients over longer periods. A special portable ECG system, designed in 1961 by N.J. Holter, records the cardiac activity of patients as they go about their daily activities.

The Holter monitor currently in use consists of electrodes placed on the chest wall and lower abdomen and a special portable ECG recorder. The patient can then be monitored over a long period (e.g., 24 hours). Two ECG leads are usually recorded. The tape is played back, and the P-QRS-T complexes are displayed on a special screen. Printouts of any portion of the ECG can be obtained for further study and permanent records.

Portable *patient-activated* monitors are now available to record ECGs in individuals with very intermittent symptoms. These event recorders are designed with replaceable electrodes so that patients can be monitored for several weeks as they go about their usual activities.

Review

The electrical currents produced during atrial and ventricular depolarization and repolarization are detected by electrodes placed on the extremities and chest wall; 12 leads are usually recorded:

1. The six *extremity (limb)* leads record voltages from the heart that are directed onto the frontal plane of the body. (This plane divides the body into front and back halves.) The extremity leads include three bipolar extremity leads (I, II, and III) and three augmented unipolar extremity leads (aV_R, aV_L, and aV_F).
   a. A *bipolar* lead records the difference between voltages from the heart detected at two extremities. The bipolar extremity leads can be represented by Einthoven's triangle (see Fig. 3.4). They are related by the equation II = I + III. A *unipolar* lead records voltages at one point relative to zero potential. The unipolar extremity leads can also be represented by a triaxial diagram (see Fig. 3.6). They are related by the equation $aV_R + aV_L + aV_F = 0$.

    b. The three unipolar extremity leads and the three bipolar extremity leads can be shown on the same diagram, so that the axes of all six leads intersect at a common point, producing the *hexaxial lead diagram.*

    c. As a general rule, the P-QRS-T pattern in lead I resembles that in lead aV_L. Leads aV_R and II usually show reverse patterns. Lead aV_F usually resembles lead III.

  2. The six *chest (precordial)* leads (V_1 to V_6) record voltages from the heart as directed onto the horizontal plane of the body (dividing the body into an upper and a lower half). They are taken with electrodes in specific anatomic locations (see Fig. 3.8).

    In addition to the 12 conventional leads, ECGs can be taken in special ways. Monitor leads, in which electrodes are placed on the chest, are generally used in cardiac care units (CCUs). (Fig. 3.13 shows the usual location of the chest electrodes for a monitor lead.) Continuous ECGs are often recorded with the Holter apparatus for a period of 24 or more hours in ambulatory patients who have a transient or an unpredictable arrhythmia. Sporadic symptoms can be correlated with ECG rhythm changes by using patient-activated event recorders.

Questions

1. Leads I and II are shown below. Draw the P-QRS-T pattern in lead III.

2. Leads I, II, and III are shown below. What is wrong with them?

3. Draw the hexaxial lead diagram that shows the six frontal plane (extremity) leads.

4. Why does the P-QRS-T pattern in lead aV_R usually show a reverse of the pattern seen in lead II?

4

The Normal ECG

The previous chapters reviewed the cycle of atrial and ventricular depolarization and repolarization detected by the ECG as well as the 12-lead system used to record this electrical activity. This chapter describes the P-QRS-T patterns seen normally in each of the 12 leads. Fortunately, you do not have to memorize 12 or more separate patterns. Rather, if you understand a few basic ECG principles and the sequence of atrial and ventricular depolarization, you can predict the normal ECG patterns in each lead.

As the sample ECG in Fig. 3.2 showed, each of the 12 leads appears to be different. In some leads, for example, the P waves are positive (upward); in others they are negative (downward). In some leads the QRS complexes are represented by an rS wave; in other leads they are represented by RS or qR waves. Finally, the T waves are positive in some leads and negative in others. What determines this variety in the appearance of ECG complexes in the different leads, and how does the repetitive cycle of cardiac electrical activity produce such different patterns in these leads?

Three Basic "Laws" of Electrocardiography

To answer the preceding questions, you need to understand three basic ECG "laws" (Fig. 4.1):

1. A *positive (upward) deflection* appears in any lead if the wave of depolarization spreads toward the positive pole of that lead. Thus if the path of atrial stimulation is directed downward and to the patient's left, toward the positive pole of lead II, a positive (upward) P wave is seen in lead II (Figs. 4.2 and 4.3). Similarly, if the ven- tricular stimulation path is directed to the left, a positive deflection (R wave) is seen in lead I (see Fig. 4.1, *A*).

2. A *negative (downward) deflection* appears in any lead if the wave of depolarization spreads toward the negative pole of that lead (or away from the positive pole). Thus if the atrial stimulation path spreads downward and to the left, a negative P wave is seen in lead aV$_R$ (see Figs. 4.2 and 4.3). If the ventricular stimulation path is directed entirely away from the positive pole of any lead, a negative QRS complex (QS deflection) is seen (see Fig. 4.1, *B*).

3. If the mean depolarization path is directed at right angles (perpendicular) to any lead, a small *biphasic deflection* (consisting of positive and negative deflections of equal size) is usually seen. If the atrial stimulation path spreads at right angles to any lead, a biphasic P wave is seen in that lead. If the ventricular stimulation path spreads at right angles to any lead, the QRS complex is biphasic (see Fig. 4.1, *C*). A biphasic QRS complex may consist of either an RS pattern or a QR pattern.

In summary, when the mean depolarization wave spreads toward the positive pole of any lead, it produces a positive (upward) deflection. When it spreads toward the negative pole (away from the positive pole) of any lead, it produces a negative (downward) deflection. When it spreads at right angles to any lead axis, it produces a biphasic deflection.

Mention of repolarization—the return of stimulated muscle to the resting state—has deliberately been omitted. The subject is touched on later in this chapter in the discussion of the normal T wave.

Three Basic Laws of Electrocardiography

A
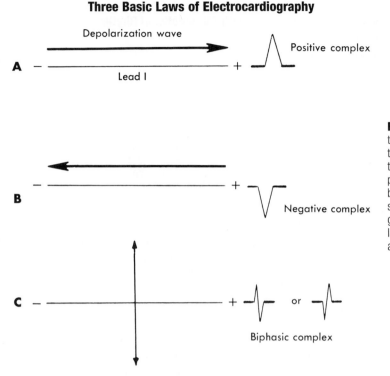

Depolarization wave

Positive complex

Lead I

B

Negative complex

C

or

Biphasic complex

Fig. 4.1 A, A positive complex is seen in any lead if the wave of depolarization spreads toward the positive pole of that lead. **B,** A negative complex is seen if the depolarization wave spreads toward the negative pole (away from the positive pole) of the lead. **C,** A biphasic (partly positive, partly negative) complex is seen if the mean direction of the wave is at right angles (perpendicular) to the lead. These three basic laws apply to both the P wave (atrial depolarization) and the QRS complex (ventricular depolarization).

Direction of Atrial Depolarization with Normal Sinus Rhythm

Fig. 4.2 With normal sinus rhythm the atrial depolarization wave *(arrow)* spreads from the right atrium downward toward the AV junction and left leg.

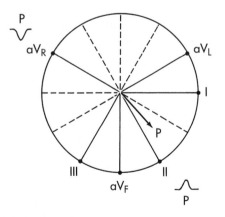

Fig. 4.3 With sinus rhythm the normal P wave is negative (downward) in lead aV$_R$ and positive (upward) in lead II. Recall that with normal atrial depolarization the arrow points down toward the patient's left (see Fig. 4.2), away from the positive pole of lead aV$_R$ and toward the positive pole of lead II.

Keeping the three ECG laws in mind, all you need to know is the direction in which depolarization spreads through the heart at any time. Using this information, you can predict what the P waves and the QRS complexes look like in any lead.

Normal P Wave

The P wave, which represents atrial depolarization, is the first waveform seen in any cycle. Atrial depolarization is initiated by the sinus node in the right atrium (see Fig. 1.1). The atrial depolarization path therefore spreads from right to left and downward toward the atrioventricular (AV) junction. The spread of atrial depolarization can be represented by an arrow* that points downward and to the patient's left (see Fig. 4.2).

Fig. 3.7, *C*, which shows the spatial relationship of the six frontal plane (extremity) leads, is redrawn in Fig. 4.3. Notice that the positive pole of lead aV_R points upward in the direction of the right shoulder. The normal path of atrial depolarization spreads downward toward the left leg (away from the positive pole of lead aV_R). *Therefore with normal sinus rhythm lead aV_R always shows a negative P wave.* Conversely, lead II is oriented with its positive pole pointing downward in the direction of the left leg (see Fig. 4.3). Therefore the normal atrial depolarization path is directed toward the positive pole of that lead. *When normal sinus rhythm is present, lead II always records a positive (upward) P wave.*

In summary, when normal sinus rhythm is present, the P wave is always negative in lead aV_R and positive in lead II.

Using the same principles of analysis, can you predict what the P wave looks like in leads II and aV_R when the heart is being paced not by the sinus node but by the AV junction (AV junctional rhythm)? When the AV junction (or an *ectopic* pacemaker in the lower part of either atrium)

---

*Because the arrows used to represent cardiac electrical potentials have both specific direction and specific magnitude, they are *vectors*. The details of *vectorcardiography* lie outside the scope of this book, although vectorial principles are used throughout the discussions.

Direction of Atrial Depolarization with AV Junctional Rhythm

Fig. 4.4 When the atrioventricular (AV) junction (or an ectopic pacemaker in the low atrial area) acts as the cardiac pacemaker (junctional rhythm), the atria are depolarized in a retrograde (backward) fashion. In this situation, an arrow representing atrial depolarization points upward toward the right atrium. The opposite of the pattern is seen with sinus rhythm.

is pacing the heart, atrial depolarization must spread up the atria in a *retrograde* direction, which is just the opposite of what happens with normal sinus rhythm. Therefore an arrow representing the spread of atrial depolarization with AV junctional rhythm points upward and to the right (Fig. 4.4), just the opposite of what occurs with normal sinus rhythm. The spread of atrial depolarization upward and to the right results in a positive P wave in lead aV_R, since the stimulus is spreading toward the positive pole of that lead (Fig. 4.5). Conversely, lead II shows a negative P wave.

AV junctional rhythms are considered in detail in Part 2. The topic is introduced in this chapter simply to show how the polarity of the P waves in lead aV_R and lead II depends on the direction of atrial depolarization and how the patterns can be predicted using simple basic principles.

At this point, you need not be concerned with the polarity of P waves in the other 10 leads. You can usually obtain all the clinical information you need to determine whether the sinus node is pacing the atria by simply looking at the P waves in leads II and aV_R. The size and shape of these waves in other leads may be important in determining

Orientation of P Waves with AV Junctional Rhythm

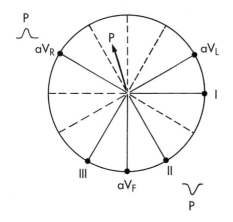

Fig. 4.5 With atrioventricular (AV) junctional rhythm (or low atrial ectopic rhythm), the P waves are upward (positive) in lead aV$_R$ and downward (negative) in lead II.

whether left or right atrial enlargement is present (see Chapter 6).

Normal QRS Complex

The principles used to predict P waves can also be applied in deducing the shape of the QRS waveform in the various leads. The QRS, which represents ventricular depolarization, is somewhat more complex than the P wave, but the same basic ECG rules apply to both.

To predict what the QRS looks like in the different leads, you must first know the direction of ventricular depolarization. Although the spread of atrial depolarization can be represented by a single arrow, the spread of ventricular depolarization consists of two major sequential phases:

1. The first phase of ventricular depolarization is of relatively brief duration (shorter than 0.04 sec) and small amplitude. It results from spread of the stimulus through the interventricular septum. The septum is the first part of the ventricles to be stimulated. Furthermore, the left side of the septum is stimulated first (by a branch of the left bundle of His). Thus depolarization spreads from the left ventricle

to the right across the septum. Phase one of ventricular depolarization (septal stimulation) can therefore be represented by a small arrow pointing from the left septal wall to the right (Fig. 4.6, *A*).

2. The second phase of ventricular depolarization involves simultaneous stimulation of the main mass of both the left and right ventricles from the inside (endocardium) to the outside (epicardium) of the heart muscle. In the normal heart the left ventricle is electrically predominant. In other words, it electrically overbalances the right ventricle. Therefore an arrow representing phase two of ventricular stimulation points toward the left ventricle (Fig. 4.6, *B*).

In summary, the ventricular depolarization process can be divided into two main phases: stimulation of the interventricular septum (represented by a short arrow pointing through the septum into the right ventricle) and simultaneous left and right ventricular stimulation (represented by a larger arrow pointing through the left ventricle and toward the left chest).

Now that the ventricular stimulation sequence has been outlined, you can begin to predict the types of QRS patterns this sequence produces in the different leads. For the moment, the discussion is limited to QRS patterns normally seen in the chest leads (the horizontal plane leads).

CHEST LEADS

As discussed in Chapter 3, lead V$_1$ shows voltages detected by an electrode placed on the right side of the sternum (fourth intercostal space). Lead V$_6$, a left chest lead, shows voltages detected in the left midaxillary line (see Fig. 3.8). What does the QRS complex look like in these leads (see Fig. 4.6)? Ventricular stimulation occurs in two phases:

1. The first phase of ventricular stimulation, septal stimulation, is represented by an arrow pointing to the right, reflecting the left-to-right spread of the depolarization stimulus through the septum (see Fig. 4.6, *A*). This small arrow points toward the positive pole of lead V$_1$. Therefore the spread of stimulation to the right during the first phase produces a small positive

Normal Ventricular Depolarization

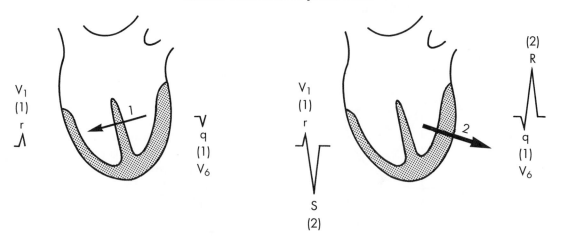

A   **B**

Fig. 4.6 A, The first phase of ventricular depolarization proceeds from the left wall of the septum to the right. An arrow representing this phase points through the septum from the left to the right side. **B,** The second phase involves depolarization of the main bulk of the ventricles. The arrow points through the left ventricle because this ventricle is normally electrically predominant. The two phases produce an rS complex in the right chest lead (V_1) and a qR complex in the left chest lead (V_6).

deflection (r wave) in lead V_1. What does lead V_6 show? The left-to-right spread of septal stimulation produces a small negative deflection (q wave) in lead V_6. Thus the same electrical event (septal stimulation) produces a small positive deflection (or r wave) in lead V_1 and a small negative deflection (q wave) in a left precordial lead, like lead V_6. (This situation is analogous to the one described for the P wave, which is normally positive in lead II but always negative in lead aV_R.)

2. The second phase of ventricular stimulation is represented by an arrow pointing in the direction of the left ventricle (Fig. 4.6, *B*). This arrow points away from the positive pole of lead V_1 and toward the negative pole of lead V_6. Therefore the spread of stimulation to the left during the second phase results in a negative deflection in the right precordial leads and a positive deflection in the left precordial leads. Lead V_1 shows a deep negative (S) wave, and lead V_6 displays a tall positive (R) wave.

In summary, with normal QRS patterns, lead V_1 shows an rS type of complex. The small initial

r wave represents the left-to-right spread of septal stimulation. This wave is sometimes referred to as the *septal r wave* because it reflects septal stimulation. The negative (S) wave reflects the spread of ventricular stimulation forces during phase two, away from the right and toward the dominant left ventricle. Conversely, viewed from an electrode in the V_6 position, septal and ventricular stimulation produce a qR pattern. The q wave is a *septal q wave*, reflecting the left-to-right spread of the stimulus through the septum away from lead V_6. The positive (R) wave reflects the leftward spread of ventricular stimulation voltages through the left ventricle.

Once again, to reemphasize, the same electrical event, whether depolarization of the atria or ventricles, produces very different looking waveforms in different leads because the spatial orientation of the leads is different.

What happens *between* leads V_1 and V_6? The answer is that as you move across the chest (in the direction of the electrically predominant left ventricle), the R wave tends to become relatively larger and the S wave becomes relatively smaller. This increase in height of the R wave, which usu-

Normal R Wave Progression

Fig. 4.7 R waves in the chest leads normally become relatively taller from lead V_1 to the left chest leads. **A,** Notice the transition in lead V_3. **B,** Somewhat delayed R wave progression, with the transition in lead V_5. **C,** Early transition in lead V_2.

ally reaches a maximum around lead V_4 or V_5, is called *normal R wave progression.* Fig. 4.7 shows examples of normal R wave progression.

At some point, generally around the V_3 or V_4 position, the ratio of the R wave to the S wave becomes 1. This point, where the amplitude of the R wave equals that of the S wave, is called the *transition zone* (see Fig. 4.7). In the ECGs of some normal people the transition may be seen as early as lead V_2. This is called *early transition.* In other cases the transition zone may not appear until leads V_5 and V_6. This is called *delayed transition.*

Examine the set of normal chest leads in Fig. 4.8. Notice the rS complex in lead V_1 and

the qR complex in lead V_6. The R wave tends to become gradually larger as you move toward the left chest leads. The transition zone, where the R wave and S wave are about equal, is in lead V_4. In normal chest leads the R wave voltage does not have to become literally larger as you go from leads V_1 and V_6. However, the overall trend should show a relative increase. In Fig. 4.8, for example, notice that the complexes in leads V_2 and V_3 are about the same and that the R wave in lead V_5 is taller than the R wave in lead V_6.

In summary, the normal chest lead ECG shows an rS-type complex in lead V_1 with a steady increase in the relative size of the R wave toward

Normal Chest Lead ECG

Fig. 4.8 The transition is in lead V$_4$. In lead V$_1$, notice the normal septal r wave as part of an rS complex. In lead V$_6$ the normal septal q is part of a qR complex.

the left chest and a decrease in S wave amplitude. Leads V$_5$ and V$_6$ generally show a qR-type complex.*

The concept of *normal R wave progression* is key in distinguishing normal and abnormal ECG patterns. For example, imagine the effect that an anterior wall MI would have on normal R wave progression. Anterior wall infarction results in the death of myocardial cells and the loss of normal positive (R wave) voltages. Therefore one major ECG sign of an anterior wall infarction is the loss of normal R wave progression in the chest leads. (see Chapters 8 and 9).

An understanding of normal R wave progression in the chest leads also provides a basis for recognizing other basic ECG abnormalities. For example, consider the effect of left or right ventricular hypertrophy (enlarged muscle mass) on the chest lead patterns. As mentioned previously, the left ventricle is normally electrically predominant and left ventricular depolarization produces deep (negative) S waves in the right chest leads with tall (positive) R waves in the left chest leads. With left ventricular hypertrophy these left ven-

tricular voltages are further increased, resulting in very tall R waves in the left chest leads and very deep S waves in the right chest leads. On the other hand, right ventricular hypertrophy shifts the balance of electrical forces to the right, producing tall positive waves (R waves) in the right chest leads (see Chapter 6).

EXTREMITY (LIMB) LEADS

Of the six extremity leads (I, II, III, aV$_R$, aV$_L$, and aV$_F$), lead aV$_R$ is the easiest to visualize. The positive pole of lead aV$_R$ is oriented upward and toward the right shoulder. The ventricular stimulation forces are oriented primarily toward the left ventricle. Therefore lead aV$_R$ normally shows a predominantly negative QRS complex. Lead aV$_R$ may display any of the QRS-T complexes shown in Fig. 4.9. In all cases the QRS is predominantly negative. The T wave in lead aV$_R$ is also normally negative.

The QRS patterns in the other five extremity leads are somewhat more complicated. The reason is that the QRS patterns in the extremity leads show considerable normal variation. For example, the extremity leads in the ECGs of some normal people may show qR-type complexes in leads I and aV$_L$ and rS-type complexes in leads III and aV$_F$ (Fig. 4.10). The ECGs of other people may show just the opposite picture, with qR complexes in leads II, III, and aV$_F$ and RS complexes in lead aV$_L$ and sometimes lead I (Fig. 4.11).

What accounts for this marked normal variability in the QRS patterns shown in the extremity leads? The patterns that are seen depend on the electrical position of the heart. The term *electrical position* is virtually synonymous with *mean QRS axis*, which is described in greater detail in Chapter 5.

In simplest terms the electrical position of the heart may be described as either *horizontal* or *vertical*:

• When the heart is electrically horizontal *(horizontal QRS axis)*, ventricular depolarization is directed mainly horizontally and to the left in the frontal plane. As the frontal plane diagram in Fig. 3.10 shows, the positive poles of leads I

---

*Normal chest lead patterns may show slight variation from the patterns discussed thus far. For example, on some normal ECGs, lead V$_1$ shows a QS pattern, not an rS pattern. In other normal chest lead patterns the septal q wave in the left chest leads may not be seen; thus leads V$_5$ and V$_6$ show an R wave and not a qR complex. On still other normal ECGs, leads V$_5$ and V$_6$ may show a narrow qRs complex as a normal variant (see Fig. 3.2, lead V$_4$) and lead V$_1$ may show a narrow rSr'.

Normal Patterns in Lead aV_R

Fig. 4.9 Lead aV_R normally shows one of three basic negative patterns: an rS complex, a QS complex, or a Qr complex. The T wave also is normally negative.

Normal Horizontal QRS Axis

Fig. 4.10 With a horizontal QRS position (axis), leads I and aV_L show qR complexes, lead II shows an RS complex, and leads III and aV_F show rS complexes.

Normal Vertical QRS Axis

Fig. 4.11 With a vertical QRS position (axis), leads II, III, and aV_F show qR complexes, but lead aV_L (and sometimes lead I) shows an RS complex. This is the reverse of the pattern that occurs with a normal horizontal axis.

and aV_L are oriented horizontally and to the left. Therefore when the heart is electrically horizontal, the QRS voltages are directed toward leads I and aV_L. Consequently, a tall R wave (usually as part of a qR complex) is seen in these leads.

- When the heart is electrically vertical *(vertical QRS axis)*, ventricular depolarization is directed mainly downward. In the frontal plane diagram (see Fig. 3.10), the positive poles of leads II, III, and aV_F are oriented downward. Therefore when the heart is electrically vertical, the QRS voltages are directed toward leads II, III, and aV_F. This produces a tall R wave (usually as part of a qR complex) in these leads.

The concepts of electrically horizontal and electrically vertical heart positions can be expressed in another way. When the heart is electrically horizontal, leads I and aV_L show qR complexes similar to the qR complexes seen normally in the left chest leads (V_5 and V_6). Leads II, III, and aV_F show rS or RS complexes similar to those seen in the right chest leads normally. Therefore when the heart is electrically horizontal, the patterns in leads I and aV_L resemble those in leads V_5 and V_6 whereas the patterns in leads II, III, and aV_F resemble those in the right chest leads. Conversely, when the heart is electrically vertical, just the opposite patterns are seen in the extremity leads. With a vertical heart, leads II, III, and aV_F show qR complexes similar to those seen in the left chest leads, and leads I and aV_L show rS-type complexes resembling those in the right chest leads.

Dividing the electrical position of the heart into vertical and horizontal variants is obviously an oversimplification. In Fig. 4.12, for example, leads I, II, aV_L, and aV_F all show positive QRS complexes. Therefore this tracing has features of *both* the vertical and the horizontal variants. (Sometimes this pattern is referred to as an "intermediate" heart position.)

For present purposes, however, you can regard the QRS patterns in the extremity leads as basically variants of either the horizontal or the vertical QRS patterns described.

In summary, the extremity leads in normal ECGs can show a variable QRS pattern. Lead aV_R normally always records a predominantly negative QRS complex (Qr, QS, or rS). The QRS patterns in the other extremity leads vary depending on the electrical position (QRS axis) of the heart. With an electrically vertical axis, leads II, III, and aV_F show qR-type complexes. With an electrically horizontal axis, leads I and aV_L show qR complexes. Therefore it is not possible to define a single normal ECG pattern; rather, there is a normal variability. Students and clinicians must familiarize themselves with the normal variants in both the chest leads and the extremity leads.

Normal ST Segment

As noted in Chapter 2, the normal ST segment, representing the early phase of ventricular repolarization, is usually isoelectric (flat on the baseline). Slight deviations (generally less than 1 mm)

Normal Intermediate QRS Axis

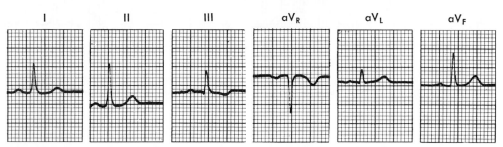

Fig. 4.12 Extremity leads sometimes show patterns that are hybrids of vertical and horizontal variants, with R waves in leads I, II, III, aV_L, and aV_F. This represents an intermediate QRS axis and is also a normal variant.

may be seen normally. As described in Chapter 10, the ECGs of certain normal people show more marked ST segment elevations as a normal variant (early repolarization pattern). Finally, examine the ST segments in the right chest leads (V_1 to V_3) of Figs. 3.2 and 6.10. Notice that they are short and the T waves appear to take off almost from the J point (junction of the QRS complex and ST segment). This pattern of an early takeoff of the T wave in the right chest leads is not an uncommon finding in normal individuals.

Normal T Wave

Ventricular repolarization—the return of stimulated muscle to the resting state—produces the ST segment, T wave, and U wave. Deciding whether the T wave in any lead is normal is generally straightforward. As a rule, the T wave follows the direction of the main QRS deflection. Thus when the main QRS deflection is positive (upright), the T wave is normally positive.

Some more specific rules about the direction of the normal T wave can be formulated. The normal T wave is always negative in lead aV_R but positive in lead II. Left-sided chest leads such as V_4 to V_6 normally always show a positive T wave.

The T wave in the other leads may be variable. In the right chest leads (V_1 and V_2) the T wave may be normally negative, isoelectric, or positive but it is almost always positive by lead V_3.* Furthermore, if the T wave is positive in any chest lead, it must remain positive in all chest leads to the left of that lead. Otherwise, it is abnormal. For example, if the T wave is negative in leads V_1 and V_2 and becomes positive in lead V_3, it should normally remain positive in leads V_4 to V_6.

The polarity of the T wave in the extremity leads depends on the electrical position of the heart. With a horizontal heart the main QRS deflection is positive in leads I and aV_L and the T wave is also positive in these leads. With an electrically vertical heart the QRS is positive in leads II, III, and aV_F and the T wave is also positive in these leads. However, on some normal ECGs with a vertical axis the T wave may be negative in lead III.

*In children and in some normal adults, a downward T wave may extend as far left as lead V_3 or V_4. This is known as the *juvenile T wave pattern.*

Review

The three basic "laws" of electrocardiography are as follows:
1. A *positive (upward) deflection* is seen in any lead if depolarization spreads toward the positive pole of that lead.
2. A *negative (downward) deflection* is seen if depolarization spreads toward the negative pole (or away from the positive pole) of any lead.
3. If the mean depolarization path is directed at right angles *(perpendicular)* to any lead, a small *biphasic (RS or QR) deflection* is seen.

Atrial depolarization starts in sinus node and spreads downward and to the patient's left, toward the positive pole of lead II and away from the positive pole of lead aV_R. Therefore with normal sinus rhythm the P wave is always positive in lead II and negative in lead aV_R.

Ventricular depolarization consists of two sequential phases:
1. The first phase is stimulation of the ventricular septum from left to right. This produces a small (septal) r wave in the right chest leads and a small (septal) q wave in the left chest leads.

2. During the second major phase of ventricular depolarization, the stimulus spreads simultaneously outward through the right and left ventricles. Because the mass of the normal left ventricle overbalances the mass of the right ventricle, the spread of depolarization through the left ventricle predominates on the normal ECG. This spread of a stimulus through the left ventricle produces a tall R wave in the left chest leads (e.g., V_5 and V_6) in association with a small initial q wave. In the right chest leads (V_1 and V_2), the stimulus produces a deep S wave associated with a small initial r wave.

Chest leads between these extreme positions show a relative increase in R wave amplitude and a decrease in S wave amplitude.

In the extremity (limb) leads the shape of the QRS complex varies with the electrical position (axis) of the heart:

1. When the heart is electrically horizontal, leads I and aV_L show a qR pattern.
2. When the heart is electrically vertical, leads II, III, and aV_F show a qR pattern.

The normal T wave generally follows the direction of the main deflection of the QRS complex in any lead. In the chest leads the T wave may normally be negative in leads V_1 and V_2. In most adults the T wave becomes positive by lead V_2 and remains positive in the left chest leads. In the extremity leads the T wave is always positive in lead II and negative in lead aV_R. When the heart is electrically horizontal, the QRS complex and T wave are positive in leads I and aV_L. When the heart is electrically vertical, the QRS complex and T wave are positive in leads II, III, and aV_F.

Questions

1. Examine the 12-lead ECG and lead II rhythm strip shown below. Then answer these questions:
   a. Is normal sinus rhythm present?
   b. In the extremity leads, is the QRS axis electrically vertical or electrically horizontal?
   c. In the chest leads, where is the transition zone?
   d. Is the PR interval normal?
   e. Is the QRS interval normal?
   f. Are the T waves in the chest leads normal?

2. On the following ECG, is sinus rhythm present?

5

Electrical Axis and Axis Deviation

Normal ECG patterns in the chest and extremity leads were discussed in Chapter 4. The general terms *horizontal heart* (or *horizontal QRS axis*) and *vertical heart* (or *vertical QRS axis*) were used to describe the normal variations in QRS patterns seen in the extremity leads. In this chapter the concept of electrical axis is refined, and methods are presented for estimating the QRS axis quickly and simply.

Mean QRS Axis: Definition

The depolarization stimulus spreads through the ventricles in different directions from instant to instant. For example, it may be directed toward lead I at one moment and toward lead III the next. The mean direction of the QRS complex, or *mean QRS electrical axis,* can also be described. If you could draw an arrow to represent the overall, or mean, direction in which the QRS complex is pointed in the frontal plane of the body, you would be drawing the electrical axis of the QRS complex. The term *mean QRS axis* therefore describes the general direction in the frontal plane toward which the QRS complex is predominantly pointed.

Since the QRS axis is being defined in the frontal plane, the QRS is being described only in reference to the six extremity leads (the six frontal plane leads). Therefore the scale of reference used to measure the mean QRS axis is the diagram of the frontal plane leads (described in Chapter 3 and depicted again in Fig. 5.1). Einthoven's triangle can easily be converted into a triaxial lead diagram by having the three axes

(leads I, II, and III) intersect at a central point (Fig. 5.1, *A*). Similarly the axes of the three unipolar extremity leads (aV_R, aV_L, and aV_F) also form a triaxial lead diagram (Fig. 5.1, *B*). These two triaxial lead diagrams can be combined to produce a hexaxial lead diagram (Fig. 5.1, *C*). You will be using this diagram to determine the mean QRS axis and describe axis deviation.

As noted in Chapter 3, each lead has a positive and negative pole (see Fig. 5.1, *C*). As a wave of depolarization spreads toward the positive pole, an upward (positive) deflection occurs. As a wave spreads toward the negative pole, a downward (negative) deflection is inscribed.

Finally, a scale is needed to determine or calculate the mean QRS axis. By convention the positive pole of lead I is said to be at 0°. All points below the lead I axis are positive, and all points above that axis are negative (Fig. 5.2). Thus toward the positive pole of lead aV_L (−30°), the scale becomes negative. Downward toward the positive poles of leads II, III, and aV_F, the scale becomes more positive (lead II at +60°, lead aV_F at +90°, and lead III at +120°).

The completed hexaxial diagram used to measure the QRS axis is shown in Fig. 5.2. By convention again, an electrical axis that points toward lead aV_L is termed *leftward* or *horizontal.* An axis that points toward leads II, III, and aV_F is *rightward* or *vertical.*

Mean QRS Axis: Calculation

In calculating the mean QRS axis, you are answering this question: In what general direction

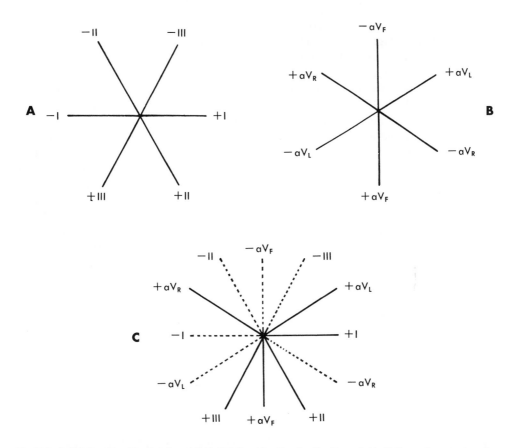

Fig. 5.1 A, Relationship of leads I, II, and III. **B,** Relationship of leads aV$_R$, aV$_L$, and aV$_F$. **C,** These diagrams have been combined to form a hexaxial lead diagram. Notice that each lead has a positive and negative pole. The negative poles are designated by dashed lines.

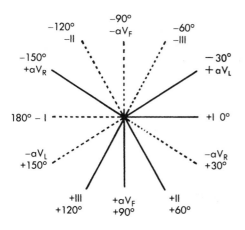

Fig. 5.2 In this hexaxial lead diagram, notice that each lead has an angular designation, with the positive pole of lead I at 0°. All leads above lead I have negative angular values, and the leads below it have positive values.

or toward which lead axis is the QRS complex predominantly oriented? In Fig. 5.3, for example, notice the tall R waves in leads II, III, and aV$_F$. These waves indicate that the heart is electrically vertical *(vertical electrical axis)*. Furthermore, the R waves are equally tall in leads II and III.* Therefore by simple inspection the mean electrical QRS axis can be seen to be directed between the positive poles of leads II and III and toward the *positive pole* of lead aV$_F$ (+90°).

As a general rule, *the mean QRS axis points midway between any two leads that show tall R waves of equal height.*

In Fig. 5.3 the mean electrical axis could have been calculated a second way. Recall from Chap-

ter 3 that if a wave of depolarization is oriented at right angles to any lead axis, a biphasic complex (RS or QR) is recorded in that lead. Reasoning in a reverse manner, if you find a biphasic complex in any of the extremity leads, the mean QRS axis must be directed at 90° to that lead. Now look at Fig. 5.3 again. Do you see any biphasic QRS complexes? Obviously lead I is biphasic and shows an RS pattern. Therefore the mean electrical axis must be directed at right angles to lead I. Since lead I on the hexaxial lead scale is at 0°, the mean electrical axis must be at right angles to 0° or at either −90° or +90°. If the axis were −90°, the depolarization forces would be oriented away from the positive pole of lead aV$_F$ and that lead would show a negative complex. In Fig. 5.3, lead aV$_F$ shows a positive complex (tall R wave); therefore the axis must be +90°.

---

*In Fig. 5.3, three leads (II, III, and aV$_F$) have R waves of equal height. In this situation the electrical axis points toward the middle lead (i.e., toward lead aV$_F$ or at +90°).

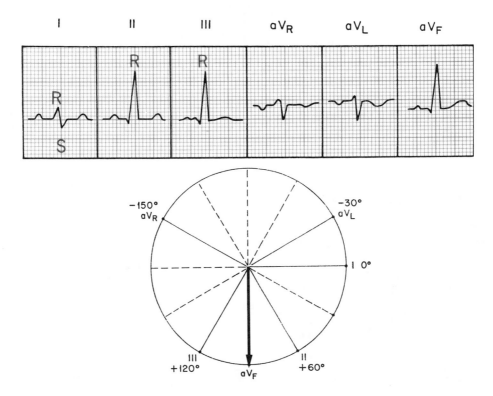

Fig. 5.3 Mean QRS axis of +90° (see text).

Fig. 5.4 presents another example. By inspection the mean QRS axis is obviously horizontal, since leads I and aV$_L$ are positive and leads II, III, and aV$_F$ are predominantly negative. The precise electrical axis can be calculated by looking at lead II, which shows a biphasic RS complex. Therefore the axis must be at right angles to lead II. Because lead II is at +60° on the hexaxial scale (see Fig. 5.2), the axis must be either −30° or +150°. If it were +150°, leads II, III, and aV$_F$ would be positive. Clearly the axis is −30°.

Another example is given in Fig. 5.5. The QRS complex is positive in leads II, III, and aV$_F$. Therefore the axis is relatively vertical. Because the R waves are of equal magnitude in leads I and III, the mean QRS axis must be oriented between these two leads, or at +60°.

Alternatively, in Fig. 5.5 the QRS axis can be calculated by looking at lead aV$_L$, which shows a biphasic RS-type complex. The axis must be at right angles to lead aV$_L$ (−30°); that is, it must be oriented at either −120° or +60°. Obviously the axis is at +60°. The electrical axis must be oriented toward lead II, which shows a tall R wave.

A second general rule can now be given: *The mean QRS axis is oriented at right angles to any lead showing a biphasic complex. In this situation the mean QRS axis points in the direction of leads showing tall R waves.*

Still another example is provided in Fig. 5.6. The electrical axis is seen to be oriented away from leads II, III, and aV$_F$ and toward leads aV$_R$ and aV$_L$, which show positive complexes. Because the R waves are of equal magnitude in leads aV$_R$ and aV$_L$, the axis must be oriented precisely between these leads, or at −90°. Alternatively, look at lead I, which shows a biphasic RS complex. In this case the axis must be directed at right angles

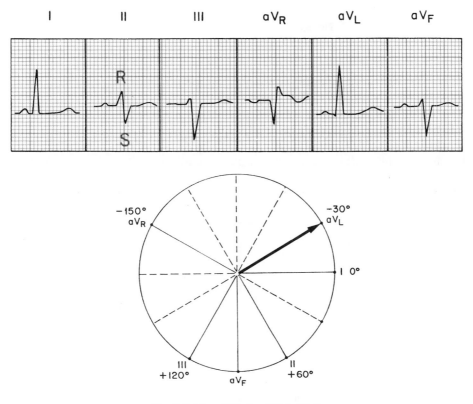

Fig. 5.4 Mean QRS of −30° (see text).

Fig. 5.5 Mean QRS axis of +60° (see text).

Fig. 5.6 Mean QRS axis of −90° (see text).

to lead I (0°); that is, it must be either −90° or +90°. Because the axis is oriented away from the positive pole of lead aV$_F$ and toward the negative pole of that lead, it must be −90°.

Again, look at Fig. 5.7. Because lead aV$_R$ shows a biphasic RS-type complex, the electrical axis must be at right angles to the axis of that lead. The axis of aV$_R$ is at −150°; therefore the electrical axis in this case must be either −60° or +120°. Clearly it is −60° because lead aV$_L$ is positive and lead III shows a negative complex.*

These basic examples should establish the ground rules for calculating the mean QRS axis. However, such calculations are generally only an

estimate or a near approximation. An error of 10° or 15° is not clinically significant. Thus it is perfectly acceptable to calculate the axis from leads in which the QRS complex is nearly biphasic or from two leads in which the R (or S) waves are of approximately equal amplitude.*

In summary, the mean QRS axis can be determined on the basis of one or both of the following rules:

---

*In Fig. 5.7 the QRS axis can also be calculated by looking at lead I, which shows an R wave of equal amplitude with the S wave in lead II. The mean QRS axis must be oriented between the positive pole of lead I (0°) and the negative pole of lead II (−120°). Therefore the axis must be at −60°.

---

*For example, when the R (or S) waves in two leads have similar but not identical voltages, the mean QRS axis does not lie exactly between these two leads. Instead, it points more toward the lead with the larger amplitude. Similarly, if a lead shows a biphasic (RS or QR) deflection with the R and S (or Q and R) waves *not* of identical amplitude, the mean QRS axis does *not* point exactly perpendicular to that lead. If the R wave is larger than the S (or Q) wave, the axis points slightly less than 90° away from the lead. If the R wave is smaller than the S (or Q) wave, the axis points slightly more than 90° away from that lead.

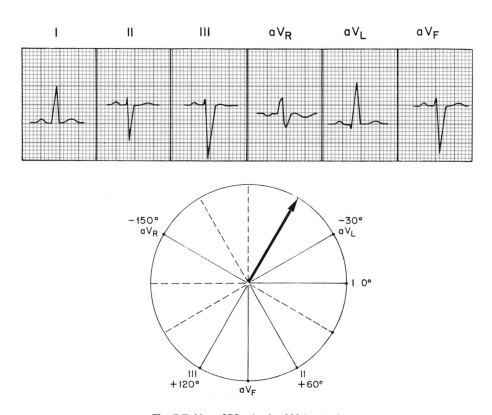

Fig. 5.7 Mean QRS axis of −60° (see text).

- The mean QRS axis points midway between the axes of two extremity leads that show tall R waves of equal amplitude.
- The mean QRS axis points at 90° (right angles) to any extremity lead that shows a biphasic (QR or RS) complex and in the direction of leads that show relatively tall R waves.

Axis Deviation

The mean QRS axis is a basic measurement that should be made on every ECG. In the ECGs of most normal people this axis lies between −30° and +100°. An axis of −30° or more negative is described as *left axis deviation (LAD)*, and one that is +100° or more positive is termed *right axis deviation (RAD)*. In other words, LAD is an abnormal extension of the mean QRS axis found in persons with an electrically horizontal heart, and RAD is an abnormal extension of the mean QRS axis in persons with an electrically vertical heart.

The mean QRS axis is determined by the anatomic position of the heart and the direction in which the stimulus spreads through the ventricles (i.e., the direction of ventricular depolarization):

1. The influence of *cardiac anatomic position* on the electrical axis can be illustrated by the effects of respiration. When a person breathes in, the diaphragm descends and the heart becomes more vertical in the chest cavity. This change

generally shifts the QRS electrical axis vertically (to the right). (Patients with emphysema and chronically hyperinflated lungs usually have anatomically vertical hearts and electrically vertical QRS axes.) Conversely, when the person breathes out, the diaphragm ascends and the heart assumes a more horizontal position in the chest. This generally shifts the QRS electrical axis horizontally (to the left).

2. The influence of the *direction of ventricular depolarization* can be illustrated by left anterior hemiblock, in which the spread of stimuli through the more superior and leftward portions of the left ventricle is delayed and the mean QRS axis shifts to the left (see Chapter 7). By contrast, with right ventricular hypertrophy (RVH) the QRS axis shifts to the right.

Recognition of RAD and LAD is quite simple:

1. *RAD exists if the QRS axis is found to be +100° or more positive.* Recall that when leads II and III show tall R waves of equal height, the QRS axis must be +90°. As an approximate rule, *if leads II and III show tall R waves and the R wave in lead III exceeds the R wave in lead II, RAD is present.* In addition, lead I shows an RS pattern with the S wave deeper than the R wave is tall (see Figs. 5.8 and 5.10).

2. *LAD exists if the QRS axis is found to be −30° or more negative.* In the ECG shown in Fig. 5.4 the QRS axis is exactly −30°. Notice that lead II shows

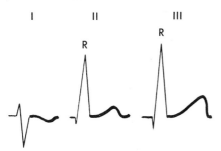

Fig. 5.8 Right axis deviation (mean QRS axis more positive than +100) can be determined by inspecting leads I, II, and III. Notice that the R wave is taller in lead III than in lead II.

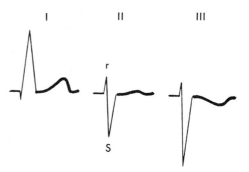

Fig. 5.9 Left axis deviation (mean QRS axis more negative than −30°) can be determined by simple inspection of leads I, II, and III. Notice that lead II shows an rS complex (with the S wave of greater amplitude than the r wave).

a biphasic (RS) complex. Remember that the location of lead II is aligned at +60° (see Fig. 5.2) and a biphasic complex indicates that the electrical axis must be at right angles to that lead (at either −30° or +150°). Thus with an axis of −30°, lead II shows an RS complex with the R and S waves of equal amplitude. *If the electrical axis is more negative than −30° (LAD), lead II shows an RS complex with the S wave deeper than the R wave is tall* (Figs. 5.9 and 5.11).

The rules for recognizing QRS axis deviation can be summarized as follows:

- RAD is present if the R wave in lead III is taller than the R wave in lead II. Notice that with RAD, lead I shows an RS-type complex in which the S wave is deeper than the R wave is tall (see Figs. 5.8 and 5.10).
- LAD is present if lead I shows a tall R wave, lead III shows a deep S wave, and lead II shows either a biphasic RS complex (with the amplitude of

the S wave exceeding the height of the R wave) (see Figs. 5.9 and 5.11) or a QS complex. Leads I and aV$_L$ both show R waves.

In Chapter 3 the terms *electrically vertical* and *electrically horizontal* heart positions (mean QRS axes) were introduced. This chapter has added the terms *left axis deviation* and *right axis deviation*. What is the difference between these terms? Electrically vertical and electrically horizontal heart positions are qualitative. With an electrically vertical mean QRS axis, leads II, III, and aV$_F$ show tall R waves. With an electrically horizontal mean QRS axis, leads I and aV$_L$ show tall R waves. With an electrically vertical heart, the actual mean QRS axis may be normal (e.g., +80°) or abnormally rightward (e.g., +120°). Similarly, with an electrically horizontal heart the actual axis may be normal (0°) or abnormally leftward (−50°).

RAD therefore is simply an extreme form of a vertical mean QRS axis, and LAD is an extreme

Right Axis Deviation

Fig. 5.10 Notice the R waves in leads II and III, with the R wave in lead III being larger than the one in lead II, from a patient with right axis deviation.

Left Axis Deviation

Fig. 5.11 Notice the rS complex in lead II, from a patient with left axis deviation.

form of a horizontal mean QRS axis. Saying that a patient has an electrically vertical or horizontal mean QRS axis does not, in fact, tell whether actual axis deviation is present.

AXIS DEVIATION: INSTANT RECOGNITION

For beginning students, precise calculation of the QRS axis is not as important as answering the following key questions: Is the QRS axis normal, or is LAD or RAD present? The answers can be obtained by inspecting the QRS complex from leads I and II (Fig. 5.12). If the area under the QRS complex in both leads is positive, the axis must be normal. If the QRS complex is predominantly positive in lead I and negative in lead II, LAD is present. If the QRS complex is predominantly negative in lead I and positive in lead II, RAD (or at least borderline RAD) is present.

CLINICAL SIGNIFICANCE

Axis deviation may be encountered in a variety of settings. RAD, with a mean QRS axis $+100°$ or more, is sometimes seen in the ECGs of normal hearts. However, RVH is an important cause of

RAD (see Chapter 6). Another cause is myocardial infarction of the lateral wall of the left ventricle. In this setting, loss of the normal leftward depolarization forces may lead "by default" to a rightward axis (see Fig. 8.11). Left posterior hemiblock is a much rarer cause of RAD (see Chapter 7). The ECGs of patients with chronic lung disease (emphysema or chronic bronchitis) often show RAD. Finally, a sudden shift in the mean QRS axis to the right (not necessarily causing actual RAD) may occur with acute pulmonary embolism (see Chapters 10 and 22).

LAD, with a mean QRS axis of $-30°$ or more, is also seen in several settings. Patients with left ventricular hypertrophy (LVH) sometimes but not always have LAD (see Chapter 6). Left anterior hemiblock is a fairly common cause of marked deviation (more negative than $-45°$). LAD may be seen in association with left bundle branch block (see Chapter 7). It may also occur in the absence of apparent cardiac disease.

However, RAD or LAD is not necessarily a sign of significant underlying heart disease. Nevertheless, its recognition (Fig. 5.12 and 5.13) often pro-

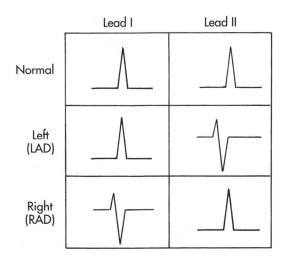

Fig. 5.12 Simple method for telling whether the QRS axis is normal using leads I and II. (*LAD,* left axis deviation; *RAD,* right axis deviation.)

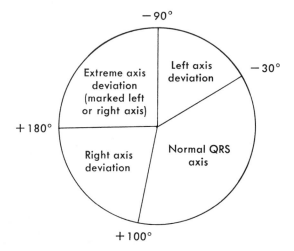

Fig. 5.13 Normal QRS axis and axis deviation. Most ECGs show either a normal axis or left or right axis deviation. Occasionally the QRS axis is between $-90°$ and $180°$. Such an extreme shift may be caused by marked left or right axis deviation.

vides supportive evidence for LVH or RVH, ventricular conduction disturbance (left anterior or posterior hemiblock), or another disorder (see Chapter 22).

Finally, the limits for LAD and RAD ($-30°$ to $+100°$) used in this book are necessarily arbitrary. Some authors use different criteria (e.g., $0°$ to $+90°$). These apparent discrepancies reflect the important fact that no absolute parameters have been established in clinical electrocardiography—only general criteria can be applied. The same problems will be encountered in the discussion of LVH and RVH (see Chapter 6) because different voltage criteria have been described by various authors.

On rare occasions, all six extremity leads show biphasic (QR or RS) complexes, which makes it impossible to calculate the mean frontal plane QRS axis. In such cases the term *indeterminate axis* is used (Fig. 5.14). An indeterminate QRS axis may occur as a normal variant, or it may be seen in a variety of pathologic settings.

Mean Electrical Axis of the P Wave and T Wave

To this point, only the mean electrical axis of the QRS complex in the frontal plane has been considered. The same principles can be applied to the mean electrical axes of the P wave and T wave in the frontal plane.

For example, when sinus rhythm is present, the normal P wave is always negative in lead aV_R and positive in lead II. Normally, therefore, the P wave is generally directed toward the positive pole of lead II (see Fig. 4.3), which makes the normal mean P wave axis about $+60°$. On the other hand, if the atrioventricular (AV) junction (and not the sinus node) is pacing the heart, the atria are stimulated in a retrograde way. When AV junctional rhythm is present, atrial depolarization spreads upward, toward lead aV_R and away from lead II (see Fig. 4.5). In this situation, lead aV_R may show a positive P wave and lead II a negative P wave, and the mean P wave axis may be about $-150°$.

The same principles can be used in calculating the mean electrical axis of the T wave in the frontal plane. As a rule the mean T wave axis and the mean QRS axis normally point in the same general (but not identical) direction. In other words, when the electrical position of the heart is horizontal, T waves normally are positive in leads I and aV_L, in association with tall R waves in those leads. When the electrical position is vertical, T waves are normally positive in leads II, III, and aV_F, in association with tall R waves in those leads. (However, the T wave is often negative in lead III normally, regardless of the electrical position of the heart.)

In summary, the concept of mean electrical axis can be applied to the QRS complex, P wave, or T wave. The mean electrical axis describes the general or overall direction of depolarization or repolarization in the frontal plane.

Fig. 5.14 Indeterminate axis. Notice the biphasic complexes (RS or QR) in all six frontal plane leads.

Review

The term *mean QRS axis* describes the general direction in which the QRS axis is pointed in the frontal plane of the body. Therefore the mean QRS axis is measured in reference to the six extremity (frontal plane) leads. These leads can be arranged in the form of a hexaxial (six axes) diagram (see Fig. 5.1, *C*).

The approximate mean QRS axis can be determined by using one of the following rules:

1. The axis will be pointed midway between the positive poles of any two leads that show R waves of equal height.
2. The axis will be pointed at right angles (perpendicular) to any lead that shows a biphasic complex and toward other leads that show tall R waves.

The normal mean QRS axis lies between $-30°$ and $+100°$. An axis more negative than $-30°$ is defined as *left axis deviation (LAD)*. An axis more positive than $+100°$ is defined as *right axis deviation (RAD)*. LAD is an extreme form of a horizontal electrical axis. RAD is an extreme form of a vertical electrical axis:

1. LAD can be readily recognized if *lead II* shows an RS complex in which the S wave is deeper than the R wave is tall. In addition, *lead I* shows a tall R wave and *lead III* shows a deep S wave. LAD is seen in the ECGs of patients with left ventricular hypertrophy, left anterior hemiblock, and certain other pathologic conditions. Sometimes it is seen in the ECGs of normal people.
2. RAD is present if the R wave in *lead III* is taller than the R wave in *lead II*. In addition, *lead I* shows an rS complex. RAD can be seen in several conditions, including right ventricular hypertrophy, lateral wall myocardial infarction, chronic lung disease, and left posterior hemiblock (see Chapter 22). In addition, RAD is sometimes seen in the ECGs of normal people.

More rarely the QRS complex is biphasic in all six extremity leads. This makes the mean electrical axis *indeterminate.*

The mean electrical axis of the P wave and T wave can be estimated in the same manner as the mean QRS axis. With normal sinus rhythm the normal P wave is about $+60°$ (positive P wave in lead II). Normally the T wave axis in the frontal plane is similar to the QRS axis. Therefore the T waves normally are positive in leads with a predominantly positive QRS complex.

Questions

1. Based on the six extremity leads (I, II, III, aV$_R$, aV$_L$, and aV$_F$) shown below, what is the approximate mean QRS axis?

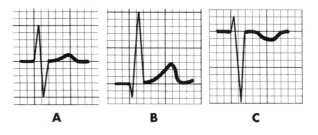

2. Tracings *A, B,* and *C* are, in mixed order, leads I, II, and III from an ECG with a mean QRS axis of $-30°$. This information should allow you to sort out which lead is which.

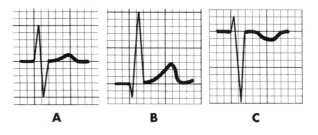

A   B   C

6

Atrial and Ventricular Enlargement

The basics of the normal ECG have been described in the first five chapters. From this point, attention is focused primarily on abnormal ECG patterns. This chapter discusses the effects on the ECG of enlargement of the four cardiac chambers.

Cardiac enlargement refers to either *dilation* of a heart chamber or *hypertrophy* of the heart muscle:

1. In dilation of a chamber the heart muscle is *stretched* and the chamber becomes enlarged. For example, with congestive heart failure (CHF) caused by acute aortic valve regurgitation, the left ventricle dilates.
2. In cardiac hypertrophy the heart muscle fibers actually *increase in size,* with resultant enlargement of the chamber. For example, aortic stenosis, which obstructs the outflow of blood from the left ventricle, leads to hypertrophy of the left ventricular muscle. Other situations (described later in this chapter) can result in hypertrophy of the atria and right ventricle. When cardiac hypertrophy occurs, the total number of heart muscle fibers does not increase; rather, each individual fiber becomes larger. One predictable ECG effect of cardiac hypertrophy is an increase in the voltage or duration of the P wave or QRS complex. Not uncommonly, hypertrophy and dilation occur together.

Both dilation and hypertrophy usually result from some type of chronic *pressure* or *volume load* on the heart muscle. The following sections discuss the ECG patterns seen with enlargement of each of the four cardiac chambers, beginning with the right atrium.

Right Atrial Abnormality

Overload of the right atrium (either dilation or actual hypertrophy) may increase the voltage of the P wave. To recognize a large P wave, you must know the dimensions of the normal P wave.

When the P wave is positive, its amplitude is measured in millimeters from the upper level of the baseline, where the P wave begins, to the peak of the wave. A negative P wave is measured from the lower level of the baseline to the lowest point of the P wave. (Measurement of the height and width of the P wave is shown in Fig. 6.1.)

Normally the P wave in every lead is less than or equal to 2.5 mm (0.25 mV) in amplitude and less than 0.12 second (three small boxes) in width. A P wave exceeding either of these dimensions in any lead is abnormal.

Overload of the right atrium may produce an abnormally tall P wave (greater than 2.5 mm). However, because pure right atrial abnormality (RAA) generally does not increase the total duration of atrial depolarization, the width of the P wave is normal (less than 0.12 second). The abnormal P wave in RAA is sometimes referred to as *P pulmonale* because the atrial enlargement that it signifies often occurs with severe pulmonary

Fig. 6.1 The normal P wave is usually no more than 2.5 mm in height and less than 0.12 second in width.

Right Atrial Abnormality (Overload)

Fig. 6.2 Tall narrow P waves may indicate right atrial abnormality or overload (P pulmonale pattern).

Right Atrial Abnormality

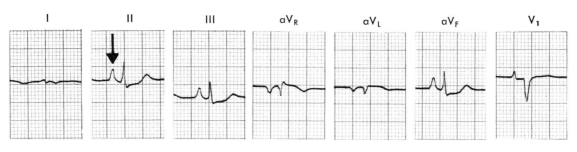

| I | II | III | aV$_R$ | aV$_L$ | aV$_F$ | V$_1$ |

Fig. 6.3 Tall P waves *(arrow)* are seen in leads II, III, aV$_F$, and V$_1$ from the ECG of a patient with chronic lung disease. This is sometimes called the *P pulmonale* pattern.

disease (Fig. 6.2). An example of RAA with a P pulmonale pattern is presented in Fig. 6.3.

The tall, narrow P waves characteristic of RAA can usually be seen best in leads II, III, aV$_F$, and sometimes V$_1$. The ECG diagnosis of P pulmonale can be made by finding a P wave exceeding 2.5 mm in any of these leads. *Echocardiographic* evidence, however, suggests that the finding of a tall, peaked P wave does not consistently correlate with RAA. On the other hand, patients may have actual right atrial overload and not tall P waves. In other words, tall peaked P waves are of limited sensitivity and specificity in the diagnosis of right atrial enlargement (see Chapter 19).

RAA is seen in a variety of clinical settings. It is usually associated with right ventricular enlargement. Two of the most common clinical causes of RAA are pulmonary disease and congenital heart disease. The pulmonary disease may be either acute (bronchial asthma, pulmonary embolism) or chronic (emphysema, bronchitis). Congenital heart lesions that produce RAA include pulmonic valve stenosis, atrial septal defects, Ebstein's anomaly (a malformation of the tricuspid valve), and tetralogy of Fallot.

Left Atrial Abnormality

Enlargement of the left atrium by dilation or actual hypertrophy also produces predictable changes in the P wave. Normally the left atrium depolarizes after the right atrium. Thus left atrial enlargement should prolong the total duration of atrial depolarization, indicated by an abnormally wide P wave. Left atrial enlargement (LAE) characteristically produces a wide P wave with a duration of 0.12 second or more (at least three small boxes). With enlargement of the left atrium the amplitude (height) of the P wave may be either normal or increased.

Some patients, particularly those with coronary artery disease, may have broad P waves without detectable enlargement of the left atrium. The abnormal P waves probably represent an atrial conduction delay in a normal-sized chamber. Therefore, rather than *left atrial enlargement* the more general term *left atrial abnormality (LAA)* is increasingly being used to describe these abnormally broad P waves.

Fig. 6.4 illustrates the characteristic P wave changes seen in LAA. As shown, the P wave sometimes has a distinctive humped or notched appearance (Fig. 6.4, *A*). The second hump corresponds to the delayed depolarization of the left atrium. These humped P waves are usually best seen in one or more of the extremity leads (Fig. 6.5). The term *P mitrale* is sometimes used to describe wide P waves seen with LAA because these waves were first described in patients with rheumatic mitral valve disease.

In patients with LAA, lead V_1 sometimes shows a distinctive biphasic P wave (see Figs. 6.4, *B*, and 6.6). This wave has a small, initial positive deflection and a prominent, wide negative deflection. The negative component is longer than 0.04 second in duration or 1 mm or more in depth. The prominent negative deflection corresponds to the delayed stimulation of the enlarged left atrium. Remember that anatomically the left atrium is situated posteriorly, up against the esophagus, whereas the right atrium lies anteriorly, against the sternum. The initial positive deflection of the P wave in lead V_1 therefore indicates right atrial depolarization, whereas the deep negative deflection is a result of left atrial depolarization voltages directed posteriorly (away from the positive pole of lead V_1).

In some cases of LAA, you may see both the broad, often humped P waves in leads I and II and the biphasic P wave in lead V_1. In other cases, only broad, notched P waves are seen. Sometimes a biphasic P wave in lead V_1 is the only ECG evidence of LAA.

Left Atrial Abnormality

Fig. 6.4 Left atrial abnormality/enlargement may produce the following: wide, sometimes notched P waves in one or more extremity leads (*P mitrale*) **(A)** and/or wide biphasic P waves in lead V_1 **(B).**

Clinically, LAA may occur in a variety of settings, including the following:
- Valvular heart disease, particularly aortic stenosis, aortic regurgitation, mitral regurgitation, and mitral stenosis.*
- Hypertensive heart disease, which causes left ventricular enlargement and eventually LAA
- Cardiomyopathies
- Coronary artery disease

The patterns of LAA and RAA are summarized schematically in Fig. 6.6. Patients with enlargement of both atria *(biatrial enlargement)* may show a combination of patterns (e.g., tall and wide P waves).

Right Ventricular Hypertrophy

Although atrial enlargement (dilation or hypertrophy) may produce prominent changes in the P wave, the QRS complex is modified primarily by ventricular *hypertrophy.* The resultant ECG effects indicate actual hypertrophy of the

---

*With mitral stenosis, valvular obstruction to the emptying of the left atrium into the left ventricle eventually results in a backup of pressure through the pulmonary vessels to the right ventricle. Therefore with advanced mitral stenosis the ECG may show a combination of LAA (or atrial fibrillation) and signs of right ventricular hypertrophy (RVH), as depicted in Fig. 19.1.

Fig. 6.5 Broad, humped P waves from the ECG of a patient with left atrial enlargement (abnormality).

Atrial Enlargement (Abnormality)

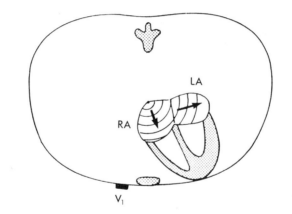

Fig. 6.6 Overload of the right atrium (*RA*) may cause tall, peaked P waves in the extremity or chest leads. An abnormality of the left atrium (*LA*) may cause broad, often notched P waves in the extremity leads and a biphasic P wave in lead V₁ with a prominent negative component representing delayed depolarization of the left atrium. (Modified from Park MK, Guntheroth WG: *How to read pediatric ECGs,* ed 3, St Louis, 1992, Mosby.)

ventricular muscle and not simply ventricular dilation.

You can predict the ECG changes produced by both right ventricular hypertrophy (RVH) and left ventricular hypertrophy (LVH) based on what you already know about normal QRS patterns. Normally the left and right ventricles depolarize simultaneously, and the left ventricle is electrically predominant because it has greater mass

(see Chapter 4). As a result, leads placed over the right side of the chest (e.g., V₁) record rS-type complexes:

In these rS-type complexes the deep negative S wave indicates the spread of depolarization volt-

QRS in Hypertrophy

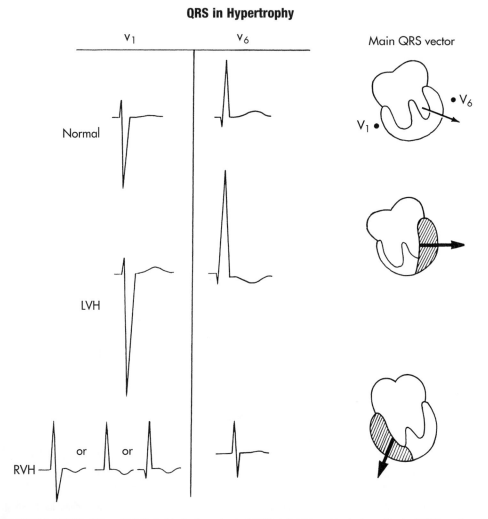

Fig. 6.7 The QRS patterns with left ventricular hypertrophy (*LVH*) and right ventricular hypertrophy (*RVH*) can be anticipated based on the abnormal physiology. Notice that left ventricular hypertrophy exaggerates the normal pattern, causing deeper right precordial S waves and taller left precordial R waves. By contrast, right ventricular hypertrophy shifts the QRS vector to the right, causing increased right precordial R waves.

ages away from the right and toward the left side. Conversely, leads placed over the left chest (e.g., V_5, V_6) record a qR-type complex:

In this complex the tall positive R wave indicates the predominant depolarization voltages that point to the left and are generated by the left ventricle.

If sufficient hypertrophy of the right ventricle occurs, the normal electrical predominance of the left ventricle can be overcome. In this situation, what type of QRS complex might you expect to see in the right chest leads? With RVH the right chest leads show tall R waves, indicating the spread of positive voltages from the hypertrophied right ventricle toward the right (Fig. 6.7). Figs. 6.8 and 6.9 show actual examples of RVH.

Instead of the rS complex normally seen in lead V_1, a tall positive (R) wave indicates marked hypertrophy of the right ventricle.

How tall does an R wave in lead V_1 have to be to make a diagnosis of RVH? In adults the normal R wave in lead V_1 is generally smaller than the S wave in that lead. An R wave exceeding the S wave in lead V_1 is suggestive but not diagnostic of RVH. Sometimes a small q wave precedes the tall R wave in lead V_1 (see Fig. 6.8).

Along with tall right chest R waves, RVH often produces two additional ECG signs: right axis deviation (RAD) and right ventricular "strain" T wave inversions (see Chapter 5).

RVH affects both depolarization (QRS complex) and repolarization (ST-T complex). For reasons not fully understood, hypertrophy of the heart muscle alters the normal sequence of repolarization. With RVH the characteristic repolarization change is the appearance of inverted T waves in the right and middle chest leads

Right Ventricular Hypertrophy

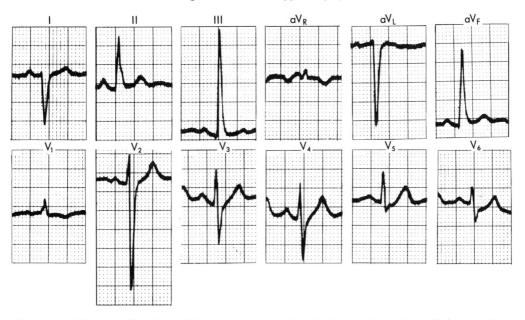

Fig. 6.8 A tall R wave with an inverted T wave caused by right ventricular strain is seen in lead V_1 from a patient with tetralogy of Fallot. Deviation of the right axis is also present. (The R wave in lead III is taller than the R wave in lead II.)

(see Figs. 6.8 and 6.9). These right chest T wave inversions are often referred to as a *right ventricular strain pattern*. ("Strain" is a descriptive term; the exact mechanism for the strain pattern is not understood.)

In summary, with RVH the ECG may show tall R waves in the right chest leads and the R wave may be taller than the S wave in lead V_1.* In addition, RAD and right precordial T wave inver-

sions are often present. Some cases of RVH are more subtle, and the ECG may show only one of these patterns. However, the appearance of all three patterns (tall right precordial R waves, RAD, and right precordial T wave inversions) firmly establishes the diagnosis of RVH.

RVH may occur in a variety of clinical settings. An important cause is congenital heart disease, such as pulmonic stenosis, atrial septal defect,*

---

*With RVH the chest leads to the left of leads showing tall R waves may display a variable pattern. Sometimes the middle and left chest leads show poor R wave progression, with rS or RS complexes all the way to lead V_6 (see Fig. 6.9). In other cases, normal R wave progression is preserved and the left chest leads also show R waves (see Fig. 6.8).

*Patients with right ventricular enlargement from the most common type of atrial septal defect often exhibit a right bundle branch block pattern (RSR' in lead V_1) with a vertical or rightward QRS axis.

Right Ventricular Hypertrophy

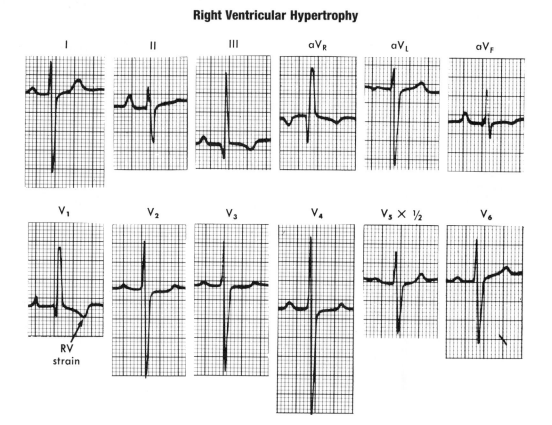

Fig. 6.9 With right ventricular hypertrophy, lead V_1 sometimes shows a tall R wave as part of the qR complex. Because of right atrial enlargement, peaked P waves are seen in leads II, III, and V_1. The T wave inversion in lead V_1 and the ST depressions in leads V_2 and V_3 are due to right ventricular overload (right ventricular [RV] *strain*). The PR interval is also prolonged (0.24 second).

tetralogy of Fallot, or Eisenmenger's syndrome. Patients with long-standing severe pulmonary disease may have pulmonary artery hypertension and RVH. As mentioned previously, mitral stenosis can produce a combination of LAA and RVH. Right ventricular strain T wave inversions in leads V_1 to V_3 may also occur without other ECG signs of RVH, as in acute pulmonary embolism (see Chapter 10).

In patients who have RVH associated with emphysema the ECG may not show any of the patterns just described. Instead of tall R waves in the right precordial leads, poor R wave progression is seen. RAD is also commonly present (see Figure 10.17).

Left Ventricular Hypertrophy

The ECG changes produced by LVH, like those from RVH, are predictable (see Fig. 6.7). Normally the left ventricle is electrically predominant over the right ventricle. As a result, prominent negative (S) waves are produced in the right chest leads, and tall positive (R) waves are seen in the left chest leads. When LVH is present, the balance of electrical forces is tipped even further to the left. Thus with LVH, abnormally tall, positive (R) waves are usually seen in the left chest leads, and abnormally deep negative (S) waves are present in the right chest leads.

The following criteria and guidelines have been established to help in the ECG diagnosis of LVH:

1. If the sum of the depth of the S wave in lead V_1 (S_{V_1}) and the height of the R wave in either lead V_5 or V_6 (R_{V_5} or R_{V_6}) exceeds 35 mm (3.5 mV), LVH should be considered (Fig. 6.10). However, high voltage in the chest leads is a common normal finding, particularly in athletic or thin young adults. Consequently, high voltage in the chest leads (S_{V_1} + R_{V_5} or R_{V_6} >35 mm) is not a *specific* indicator of LVH* (Fig. 6.11).

2. Sometimes LVH produces tall R waves in lead aV_L. An R wave of 11 to 13 mm (1.1 to 1.3 mV) or more in lead aV_L is another sign of LVH (see Fig. 6.9).* Sometimes a tall R wave in lead aV_L is the only ECG sign of LVH, and the voltage in the chest leads is normal. In other cases the chest voltages are abnormally high, with a normal R wave seen in lead aV_L.

3. Just as RVH is sometimes associated with a right ventricular strain pattern, so ST-T changes are often seen in LVH. Fig. 6.12 illustrates the characteristic shape of the ST-T complex with LVH. Notice that the complex has a distinctively asymmetric appearance, with a slight ST segment depression followed by a broadly inverted T wave. In some cases these T wave inversions are very deep. This repolarization abnormality is seen in leads with tall R waves (see Fig. 6.10).

4. With LVH the electrical axis is usually horizontal. Actual left axis deviation (i.e., an axis −30° or more negative) may also be seen. In addition, the QRS complex may become wider. Not uncommonly, patients with LVH eventually develop an incomplete or complete left bundle branch block (LBBB) pattern. Indeed, most patients with LBBB have underlying LVH (see Chapter 7).

5. Finally, the signs of LAA (broad P waves in the extremity leads or wide biphasic P waves in lead V_1) are often seen in patients with ECG evidence of LVH. Most conditions that lead to LVH ultimately produce left atrial overload as well.

In summary, the diagnosis of LVH can be made with reasonable certainty from the ECG if you find high QRS voltages and associated ST-T changes (strain pattern). In addition, signs of LAA are often present. Because high voltage in the chest or extremity leads can sometimes be seen in normal people, especially athletes and young adults, the diagnosis of LVH should not

---

*Other LVH criteria (the Cornell voltage criteria) based on voltages in leads V_3 and aV_L have recently been suggested: for men, S_{V_3} + R_{aV_L} >28 mm; for women, S_{V_3} + R_{aV_L} >20 mm.

*Occasionally, LVH develops with an electrically vertical axis. In this situation a qR pattern with a tall R wave (exceeding 20 mm) may appear in lead aV_F.

Left Ventricular Hypertrophy

Fig. 6.10 Pattern of left ventricular hypertrophy in a patient with severe hypertension. Tall voltages are seen in the chest leads and lead aV_L (R = 17 mm). A repolarization (ST-T) abnormality, sometimes referred to as a *strain* pattern, is also present in these leads. In addition, enlargement of the left atrium is indicated by a biphasic P wave in lead V_1 and a broad, notched P wave in lead II.

be made on this finding alone.* ST-T changes resulting from left ventricular overload can also occur without other evidence of LVH.

The recognition of LVH is clinically important for two reasons:

---

*The voltage criteria used in this chapter to diagnose LVH in the chest and extremity leads are by no means absolute numbers. In fact, many different criteria have been proposed.

1. Diagnostically, LVH is a clue to the presence of a potentially life-threatening pressure or volume overload state, most importantly systemic hypertension or aortic stenosis. The three major clinical conditions associated with left ventricular volume overload are aortic regurgitation, mitral regurgitation, and dilated cardiomyopathy.

2. Prognostically, patients with LVH from any cause are at increased risk for major cardiovas-

Fig. 6.11 Tall voltages in the chest leads ($R_{V_1} + S_{V_5}$ = 36 mm) from a 20-year-old man represent a common normal ECG variant, particularly in athletic or thin young adults. The ST-T complexes are normal, without evidence of repolarization (ST-T) abnormalities or left atrial abnormality.

Repolarization Abnormality with Left Ventricular Hypertrophy

Fig. 6.12 Repolarization abnormalities associated with left ventricular hypertrophy are often referred to as the *strain* pattern, an imprecise but commonly used term. Notice the characteristic wavy ST-T pattern with T wave inversion in the leads that show tall R waves.

cular complications, including CHF and serious atrial or ventricular arrhythmias.

The ECG in Cardiac Enlargement: A Perspective

The ECG findings associated with enlargement of each of the four cardiac chambers have been presented. In some cases, combined patterns are seen on the same tracing (e.g., LAA and RVH in mitral stenosis, LAA and LVH in systemic hypertension). If hypertrophy is present in both ventricles, the ECG usually shows mainly evidence of LVH. Another pattern that may provide an important clue to biventric-

ular hypertrophy is LVH with right axis deviation.

Always remember that in the assessment of cardiac size, the ECG is only an indirect laboratory test and not an absolute measurement. A person may have underlying cardiac enlargement that does not show up on the ECG. Conversely, the ECG may show high voltage in a normal person who does not have cardiac enlargement. When the presence or degree of cardiac chamber enlargement must be determined with more precision, an *echocardiogram* should be obtained.*

_____

*The diagnostic limitations of the ECG are discussed further in Chapter 19.

Review

Cardiac *dilation* refers to the stretching of muscle fibers, with enlargement of one or more of the cardiac chambers. Cardiac *hypertrophy* refers to an abnormal increase in the actual size of the heart muscle fibers. The ECG can indicate either right or left atrial dilation or hypertrophy but generally only right or left ventricular hypertrophy.

Right atrial abnormality (RAA), or right atrial overload, may be associated with tall peaked P waves exceeding 2.5 mm in height. These waves are usually best seen in leads II, III, aV_F, and sometimes V_1 or V_2.

Left atrial abnormality (LAA), or left atrial enlargement, is manifested by wide, sometimes notched P waves of 0.12 second or more duration in one or more of the extremity leads. A biphasic P wave with a prominent wide negative deflection may be seen in lead V_1.

Right ventricular hypertrophy may produce any or all of the following:
   1. A tall R wave in lead V_1, equal to or larger than the S wave in that lead
   2. Often, right axis deviation
   3. A right ventricular *strain* pattern (T wave inversions in the right to middle chest leads)
With left ventricular hypertrophy (LVH), any or all of the following may occur:
   1. The voltage of the S wave in lead V_1 plus the voltage of the R wave in lead V_5 or V_6 often exceeds 35 mm (S_{V_1} + R_{V_5} or R_{V_6} >35 mm).
   2. A high-voltage R wave (11 to 13 mm or more) is seen in lead a V_1 when the heart is electrically horizontal. (When the axis is vertical, lead aV_F may show a tall R wave [greater than 20 mm] as part of a qR complex.)
   3. Repolarization abnormalities include inverted T waves in leads with a qR pattern (strain pattern).
   4. Concomitant findings often include LAA, left axis deviation, and left ventricular conduction delay (wide QRS), which may lead to incomplete or complete left bundle branch block.

The diagnosis of LVH should *not* be made solely on the basis of high voltage in the chest leads because these high voltages may occur normally, particularly in young adults and thin individuals. In addition, enlargement of any of the four cardiac chambers can be present *without* diagnostic ECG changes.

Questions

1. Examine the ECG shown below:
   a. What is the heart rate?
   b. Name two abnormal findings.

7

Ventricular Conduction Disturbances

Bundle branch blocks

*R*ecall that in the normal process of ventricular activation the electrical stimulus reaches the ventricles from the atria by way of the atrioventricular (AV) junction (see Chapter 4). The first part of the ventricles to be stimulated (depolarized) is the left side of the ventricular septum. Soon after, the depolarization spreads to the main mass of the left and right ventricles by way of the left and right bundle branches. Normally the entire process of ventricular depolarization is completed within about 0.1 second (100 msec). This is the reason the normal width of the QRS complex is less than or equal to 100 msec (two and a half small boxes on the ECG graph paper). Any process that interferes with the normal stimulation of the ventricles may prolong the QRS width. This chapter focuses on the effects that blocks within the bundle branch system have on the QRS complex.

Right Bundle Branch Block

Consider, first, the effect of cutting the right bundle branch, or markedly slowing conduction in this structure. Obviously, right ventricular stimulation will be delayed and the QRS complex will be widened. The shape of the QRS with a right bundle branch block (RBBB) can be predicted on the basis of some familiar principles.

Normally the first part of the ventricles to be depolarized is the interventricular septum (see Fig. 4.6, *A*). The left side of the septum is stimulated first (by a branch of the left bundle). On the normal ECG, this septal depolarization produces a small septal r wave in lead V_1 and a small septal q wave in lead V_6 (Fig. 7.1, *A*). Clearly, RBBB should not affect the septal phase of ventricular stimulation because the septum is stimulated by a part of the left bundle.

The *second* phase of ventricular stimulation is the simultaneous depolarization of the left and right ventricles (see Fig. 4.6, *B*). RBBB should not affect this phase either, since the left ventricle is normally electrically predominant, producing deep S waves in the right chest leads and tall R waves in the left chest leads (Fig. 7.1, *B*). The change in the QRS complex produced by RBBB is a result of the delay in the total time needed for stimulation of the right ventricle. This means that after the left ventricle has completely depolarized, the right ventricle continues to depolarize.

This delayed right ventricular depolarization produces a *third* phase of ventricular stimulation. The electrical voltages in the third phase are directed to the right, reflecting the delayed depolarization and slow spread of the depolarization wave outward through the right ventricle. Therefore a lead placed over the right side of the chest (e.g., lead V_1) records this phase of ventricular stimulation as a positive wide deflection (R′ wave). The rightward spread of the delayed and slow right ventricular depolariza-

Right Bundle Branch Block

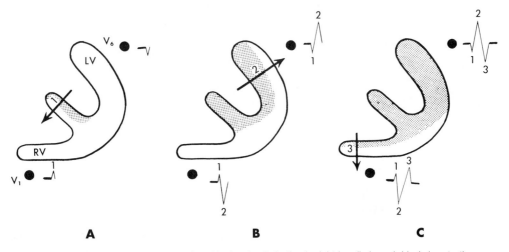

Fig. 7.1 Step-by-step sequence of ventricular depolarization in right bundle branch block (see text).

tion voltages produces a wide negative (S wave) deflection in the left chest leads (e.g., lead V_6) (Fig. 7.1, *C*).

Based on an understanding of this step-by-step process, the pattern seen in the chest leads with RBBB can be derived. With RBBB, lead V_1 shows an rSR′ complex with a broad R wave. Lead V_6 shows a qRS-type complex with a broad S wave. The tall wide R wave in the right chest leads and the deep terminal S wave in the left chest leads represent the same event viewed from opposite sides of the chest—the slow spread of delayed depolarization voltages through the right ventricle.

To make the initial diagnosis of RBBB, look at leads V_1 and V_6 in particular. The characteristic appearance of QRS complexes in these leads makes the diagnosis simple. (Fig. 7.1 shows how the delay in ventricular depolarization with RBBB produces the characteristic ECG patterns.)

In summary, the ventricular stimulation process in RBBB can be divided into three phases. The first two phases are normal septal and left ventricular depolarization. The third phase is delayed stimulation of the right ventricle. These

three phases of ventricular stimulation with RBBB are represented on the ECG by the triphasic complexes seen in the chest leads:

- Lead V_1 shows an rSR′ complex with a wide R′ wave.
- Lead V_6 shows a qRS pattern with a wide S wave.

With an RBBB the QRS complex in lead V_1 generally shows an rSR′ pattern (Fig. 7.2). Occasionally, however, the S wave never quite makes its way below the baseline. Consequently, the complex in lead V_1 has the appearance of a large notched R wave (Fig. 7.3).

Figs. 7.2 and 7.3 are typical examples of RBBB. Do you notice anything abnormal about the ST-T complexes in these tracings? If you look carefully, you can see that the T waves in the right chest leads are inverted. T wave inversions in the right chest leads are a characteristic finding with RBBB. These inversions are referred to as *secondary changes* because they reflect just the delay in ventricular stimulation. By contrast, *primary T wave abnormalities* reflect an actual change in repolarization, independent of any QRS change. Examples of primary T wave abnormalities include T wave inversions resulting from ischemia (see Chapters 8 and 9), hypokalemia

Right Bundle Branch Block

Fig. 7.2 Instead of the classic rSR′ pattern with right bundle branch block, the right precordial leads sometimes show a wide notched R wave (seen here in leads V_1 to V_3). Notice the *secondary* T wave inversions in leads V_1 to V_3, II, III, and aV_F, all of which show rSR′-type complexes. However, the abnormal ST-T changes in leads V_4 and V_5 are *primary* because they are present in leads without an R′ wave.

Right Bundle Branch Block

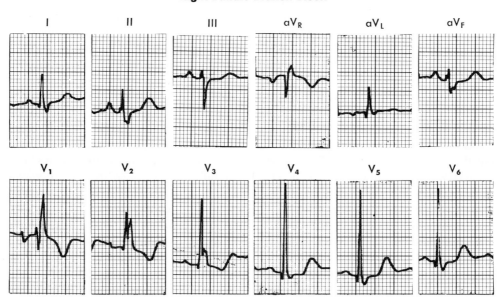

Fig. 7.3 Notice the wide rSR′ complex in lead V_1 and the qRS complex in lead V_6. Inverted T waves in the right precordial leads (in this case V_1 to V_3) are common with right bundle branch block and are called *secondary* T wave inversions.

(see Chapter 10), and drugs such as digitalis (see Chapter 10).

Some ECGs show both primary and secondary ST-T changes. In Fig. 7.3 the T wave inversions in leads V_1 to V_3 and leads II, III, and aV_F can be explained solely on the basis of the RBBB because the inversions occur in leads with an rSR′-type complex. However, the T wave inversions or ST depressions in other leads (V_4 and V_5) represent a primary change, perhaps resulting from ischemia or a drug effect.

COMPLETE AND INCOMPLETE RBBB

RBBB can be subdivided into complete and incomplete forms, depending on the width of the QRS complex. Complete RBBB is defined by a QRS that is 0.12 second or more in duration with an rSR′ in lead V_1 and a qRS in lead V_6. Incomplete RBBB shows the same QRS patterns, but its duration is between 0.1 and 0.12 second.

CLINICAL SIGNIFICANCE

RBBB may be caused by a number of factors. First, some normal people have this finding without any underlying heart disorder. Therefore RBBB itself is not necessarily abnormal. In many people, however, RBBB is associated with organic heart disease. It may occur with virtually any condition that affects the right side of the heart, including atrial septal defect with left-to-right shunting of blood, chronic pulmonary disease with pulmonary artery hypertension, and valvular lesions such as pulmonic stenosis. In some people (particularly older individuals), RBBB is related to chronic degenerative changes in the conduction system. It may also occur with acute or chronic coronary artery disease.

Pulmonary embolism, which produces acute right-sided heart overload, may cause a right ventricular conduction delay. When RBBB occurs after coronary artery bypass graft surgery, it does not seem to have any special clinical implications.

RBBB may be permanent or transient. Sometimes it appears only when the heart rate exceeds a certain critical value (rate-related RBBB).

By itself, RBBB does not require any specific treatment. However, in patients with acute ante-rior wall infarction a new RBBB may indicate an increased risk of complete heart block (see Chapter 15), particularly when the RBBB is associated with left anterior or posterior hemiblock.

Left Bundle Branch Block

Left bundle branch block (LBBB) also produces a pattern with a widened QRS complex. However, the QRS complex with LBBB is very different from that with RBBB. The major reason for this difference is that RBBB affects mainly the terminal phase of ventricular activation whereas LBBB also affects the early phase.

Recall that the first phase of ventricular stimulation—depolarization of the left side of the septum—is started by a branch of the left bundle. LBBB therefore blocks this normal pattern. When LBBB is present, the septum depolarizes from *right* to *left* and not from left to right. Thus the first major ECG change produced by LBBB is a loss of the normal septal r wave in lead V_1 and the normal septal q wave in lead V_6 (Fig. 7.4, *A*). Furthermore, the total time for left ventricular depolarization is prolonged with LBBB. As a result, the QRS complex is abnormally wide. Lead V_6 shows a wide, entirely positive (R) wave (Fig. 7.4, *B*). The right chest leads (e.g., V_1) record a negative QRS (QS) complex because the left ventricle is still electrically predominant with LBBB and therefore produces greater voltages than the right ventricle. The major change is a delay in the total time for the completion of left ventricular depolarization. Thus with LBBB the entire process of ventricular stimulation is oriented toward the left chest leads; that is, the septum depolarizes from right to left, and stimulation of the electrically predominant left ventricle is prolonged. Fig. 7.4 illustrates the sequence of ventricular activation in LBBB.*

---

*A variation of this pattern sometimes occurs: Lead V_1 may show an rS complex with a very small r wave and a wide S wave. This superficially suggests that the septum is being stimulated normally from left to right. However, lead V_6 shows an abnormally wide and notched R wave *without* an initial q wave.

Left Bundle Branch Block

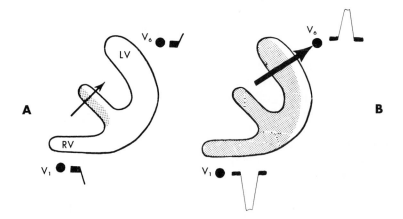

Fig. 7.4 The sequence of ventricular depolarization in left bundle branch block produces a wide QS complex in lead V₁ and a wide R wave in lead V₆.

Left Bundle Branch Block

Fig. 7.5 Notice the characteristic wide QS complex in lead V₁ and the wide R wave in lead V₆ with slight notching at the peak. The inverted T waves in leads V₅ and V₆ (secondary T wave inversions) are also characteristic of left bundle branch block.

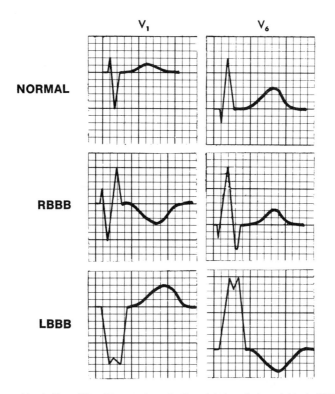

Fig. 7.6 Comparison of leads V_1 and V_6, with normal conduction, right bundle branch block *(RBBb)*, and left bundle branch block *(LBBB)*. Normally lead V_1 shows an rS complex and lead V_6 shows a qR complex. With RBBB, lead V_1 shows a wider rSR' complex and lead V_6 shows a qRS complex. With LBBB, lead V_1 shows a wide QS complex and lead V_6 shows a wide R wave.

With LBBB the QS wave in lead V_1 sometimes shows a small notching at its point, giving the wave a characteristic W shape. Similarly, the R wave in lead V_6 may show a notching at its peak, giving it a distinctive M shape. (An example of an LBBB pattern is presented in Fig. 7.5.)

Just as *secondary* T wave inversions occur with RBBB, they also occur with LBBB. As Fig. 7.5 shows, the T waves in the leads with tall R waves (e.g., the left precordial leads) are inverted; this is characteristic of LBBB. However, T wave inversions in the right precordial leads cannot be explained solely on the basis of LBBB. If present, these T wave inversions reflect some *primary* abnormality such as ischemia (see Fig. 8.21).

In summary, the diagnosis of LBBB can be made simply by inspection of leads V_1 and V_6:

- Lead V_1 usually shows a wide, entirely negative QS complex (rarely, a wide rS complex).
- Lead V_6 shows a wide, tall R wave without a q wave.

You should have no problem differentiating LBBB and RBBB patterns (Fig. 7.6). Occasionally an ECG shows wide QRS complexes that are not typical of an RBBB or LBBB pattern. In such cases the general term *intraventricular delay* is used (Fig. 7.7).

COMPLETE AND INCOMPLETE LBBB

LBBB, like RBBB, has complete and incomplete forms. With complete LBBB the QRS complex has the characteristic appearance described previously and is 0.12 second or wider. With incomplete LBBB the QRS is between 0.1 and 0.12 second wide.

Fig. 7.7 In nonspecific intraventricular conduction delay, the QRS complex is abnormally wide (0.11 second). However, such a pattern is not typical of left or right bundle branch block. In this patient the pattern was caused by an anterolateral wall myocardial infarction (see Chapter 8).

CLINICAL SIGNIFICANCE

Unlike RBBB, which is occasionally seen without evident cardiac disease, LBBB is usually a sign of organic heart disease. LBBB may develop in patients with long-standing hypertensive heart disease, a valvular lesion (e.g., calcification of the mitral annulus, aortic stenosis, or aortic regurgitation), or different types of cardiomyopathy (see Chapter 10). It is also seen in patients with coronary artery disease and often correlates with impaired left ventricular function. Most patients with LBBB have

underlying left ventricular hypertrophy (see Chapter 6). Degenerative changes in the conduction system may lead to LBBB, particularly in the elderly. Often, more than one contributing factor may be identified (e.g., hypertension and coronary artery disease). Rarely, otherwise normal individuals have an LBBB pattern without evidence of organic heart disease by examination, echocardiogram, or even invasive studies.

LBBB, like RBBB, may be permanent or transient. It also may appear only when the heart

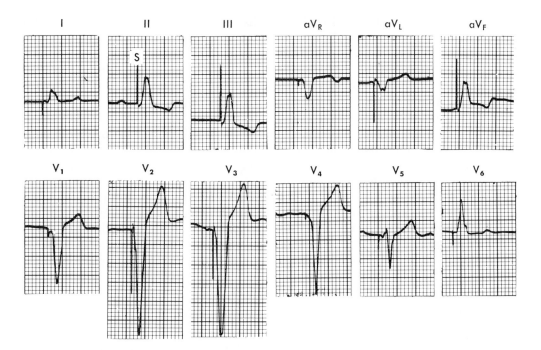

Fig. 7.8 A pacemaker inserted in the right ventricle generally produces a pattern resembling that of left bundle branch block, with a wide QS in lead V_1 and a wide R wave in lead V_6. This pattern is caused by delayed depolarization of the left ventricle. Notice the pacemaker spike in each lead preceding the QRS complex. In some leads (e.g., II) the spike *(S)* is positive; in others (V_1 to V_6), it is negative.

rate exceeds a certain critical value (rate- or acceleration-dependent LBBB).*

An important consideration is that LBBB may be the first clue to four previously undiagnosed but clinically important abnormalities: coronary artery disease, valvular heart disease, hypertensive heart disease, and cardiomyopathy.

Pacemaker Patterns

Pacemakers are battery-operated devices designed to stimulate the heart electrically. A pacemaker is used primarily when a patient's own heart rate is not adequate (e.g., in complete heart block or sick sinus syndrome). In most cases the pacemaker electrode is inserted into the right ventricle. Therefore the ECG shows an LBBB pat-

tern, which reflects delayed activation of the left ventricle.

Fig. 7.8 is an example of a pacemaker tracing. The vertical spike preceding each QRS complex is the pacemaker spike. This spike is followed by a wide QRS complex with an LBBB morphology (QS in lead V_1 with a wide R wave in lead V_6). (Pacemakers are discussed in greater detail in Chapter 20.)

Fascicular Blocks (Hemiblocks)

Fascicular blocks, or *hemiblocks,* are a slightly more complex but important topic. To this point the left bundle branch system has been described as if it were a single pathway. Actually this system has been known for many years to be subdivided into an *anterior fascicle* and a *posterior fascicle* (from the Latin *fasciculus,* meaning "small bundle"). The right bundle branch, by contrast, is a single

---

*Less commonly, LBBB occurs only when the heart decelerates below some critical value.

pathway and consists of just one main fascicle or bundle. This revised concept of the bundle branch system as a *trifascicular* highway (one right lane and two left lanes) is illustrated in Fig. 7.9.

In summary, the bundle of His divides into a right bundle branch and a left main bundle branch. The left main bundle branch then subdivides into an anterior and a posterior fascicle.

It makes sense to suppose that a block can occur at any single point (or at multiple points) in this trifascicular system. The ECG pattern with RBBB has already been presented (see Figs. 7.2 and 7.3). The pattern of LBBB can occur in one of two ways: by a block in the left main bundle before it divides or by blocks in both subdivisions (anterior and posterior fascicles).

What happens if a block occurs in just the anterior or just the posterior fascicle of the left bundle? A block in either fascicle of the left bundle branch system is called a *hemiblock* or *fascicular block*. Recognition of hemiblocks on the ECG is intimately related to the subject of axis deviation (see Chapter 5). Somewhat surprisingly, a hemiblock (unlike a full LBBB or RBBB) does not widen the QRS complex markedly. Experiments

have shown that the main effect of cutting these fascicles is a change in the QRS axis. Specifically, *left anterior* fascicular block results in marked left axis deviation ($-45°$ or more); *left posterior* fascicular block produces marked right axis deviation ($+120°$ or more).*

In summary, hemiblocks are partial blocks in the left bundle branch system and involve either the anterior or posterior fascicle. The diagnosis of a hemiblock is made from the mean QRS axis in the extremity (frontal plane) leads. This is in contrast to the diagnosis of complete (or incomplete) RBBB or LBBB, which is made primarily from the QRS patterns in the chest (horizontal plane) leads. Complete bundle branch blocks, unlike hemiblocks, do not cause a characteristic shift in the mean QRS axis.

---

*Left anterior hemiblock shifts the QRS axis to the left by delaying activation of the more superior and leftward portions of the left ventricle. Left posterior hemiblock shifts it to the right by delaying activation of the more inferior and rightward portions of the left ventricle. In both cases the QRS axis therefore is shifted *toward* the direction of delayed activation.

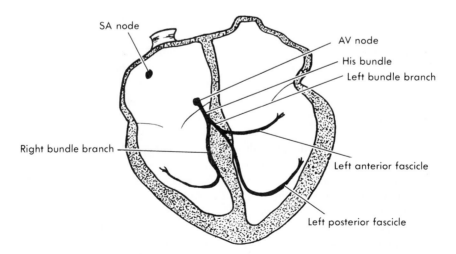

Fig. 7.9 With a trifascicular conduction system, notice that the left bundle branch subdivides into a left anterior fascicle and a left posterior fascicle. This diagram is a revision of the original drawing of the conduction system (see Fig. 1.1) (*SA,* sinoatrial; *AV,* atrioventricular).

LEFT ANTERIOR FASCICULAR BLOCK

Isolated left anterior fascicular block is diagnosed by finding a mean QRS axis of −45° or more and a QRS width of less than 0.12 second. A mean QRS axis of −45° or more can be easily recognized because the S wave in lead aV_F equals or exceeds the R wave in lead I (Fig. 7.10).* Lead aV_L usually shows a qR complex, with rS complexes in leads II, III, and aV_F (or QS waves if an inferior myocardial infarction is also present).

LEFT POSTERIOR FASCICULAR BLOCK

Isolated left fascicular block (see Fig. 9.8, *B*) is diagnosed by finding a mean QRS axis of +120° or more, with a QRS width of less than 0.12 second. Usually an rS complex is seen in lead I, and a qR complex is seen in leads II, III, and aV_F. *However, the diagnosis of left posterior fascicular block can be considered only after other, more common causes of right axis deviation (RAD) have been excluded* (see Chapter 22). These causes can include right ventricular hypertrophy (RVH), normal variant, emphysema, lateral wall infarction (see Fig. 8.11), and pulmonary embolism.

Although left anterior fascicular block is relatively common, isolated left posterior fascicular block is very rare. (Most often it occurs with RBBB.) In general, the finding of isolated left anterior fascicular blocks is not of much clinical significance. (Hemiblocks and *bifascicular* and *trifascicular* blocks are considered fur-

---

*Some authors use an axis of −30° or more negative. The original description of this pattern used a cut-off of −45° or more negative.

ther in the discussion of complete heart block in Chapter 15.)

Diagnosis of Hypertrophy in the Presence of Bundle Branch Blocks

The ECG diagnosis of hypertrophy (see Chapter 6) in the presence of bundle branch blocks may pose special problems. A few general guidelines are helpful.

When RVH occurs with RBBB, RAD is often present. A tall peaked P wave with RBBB should also suggest underlying RVH.

The usual voltage criteria for left ventricular hypertrophy (LVH) can be used in the presence of RBBB. Unfortunately, RBBB often masks these typical voltage increases.

The finding of LBBB, regardless of the QRS voltage, is highly suggestive of underlying LVH. Finding LBBB with prominent QRS voltages *and* evidence of left atrial abnormality virtually ensures the diagnosis of LVH (see Chapter 6).

Finally, it should be emphasized that the *echocardiogram* is much more accurate than the ECG in the diagnosis of cardiac enlargement (see Chapter 6).

Diagnosis of Myocardial Infarction in the Presence of Bundle Branch Blocks

The ECG diagnosis of myocardial infarction in the presence of bundle branch blocks is discussed in Chapter 8.

Fig. 7.10 Left anterior hemiblock. Notice the marked left axis deviation without significant widening of the QRS duration. Compare this with Fig. 9.8, *B*, which shows left posterior hemiblock.

Review

Right bundle branch block (RBBB) shows the following characteristic patterns: an rSR′ with a prominent wide final R′ wave in lead V_1, a qRS with a wide final S wave in lead V_6, and a QRS width of 0.12 second (three small time boxes) or more. *Incomplete RBBB* shows the same chest lead patterns, but the QRS width is between 0.1 and 0.12 second.

Left bundle branch block (LBBB) shows the following characteristic patterns: a deep wide QS (occasionally an rS with a wide S wave) in lead V_1, a prominent (often notched) R wave *without* a preceding q wave in lead V_6, and a QRS width of 0.12 second or more. *Incomplete LBBB* shows the same chest lead patterns as LBBB, but the QRS width is between 0.1 and 0.12 second.

Pacemaker patterns produced by an electrode in the right ventricle generally resemble LBBB but have a pacemaker spike before each QRS complex.

Hemiblocks (fascicular blocks) can occur because the left bundle splits into two subdivisions *(fascicles):* the left anterior fascicle and the left posterior fascicle. Conduction through either or both of these bundles can be blocked.

Left anterior fascicular block or *hemiblock* is characterized by a mean QRS axis of −45° or more. (When the mean QRS axis is −45°, left axis deviation is present and the height of the R wave in lead I [R_I] is equal to the depth of the S wave in lead aV_F [S_{aV_F}]. When the mean QRS axis is more negative than −45°, S_{aV_F} becomes larger than R_I.)

Left posterior fascicular block or *hemiblock* is characterized by marked right axis deviation (RAD). However, before the diagnosis of left posterior hemiblock is made, other more common causes of RAD must be excluded, including right ventricular hypertrophy, lateral wall infarction, chronic lung disease, and normal variants (see Chapter 22).

Questions

1. Draw the shape of the QRS complexes in leads V_1 and V_6 that would be expected with right and left bundle branch blocks.
2. Examine the chest leads shown below and then answer these questions:
   a. What is the approximate QRS width?
   b. What conduction disturbance is present?
   c. Why are the T waves in leads V_1 to V_3 inverted?

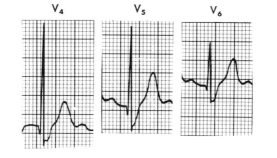

3. Examine the following 12-lead ECG and lead II rhythm strip carefully. Can you identify the major conduction abnormality?

4. Define the terms *primary* and *secondary* T wave abnormality.

True or false *(Questions 5 to 7):*

5. Left anterior hemiblock does not markedly widen the QRS complex.
6. Left bundle branch block is generally seen in patients with organic heart disease.
7. Bundle branch blocks may occur transiently.

8

Myocardial Ischemia and Infarction, Section I

Transmural ischemia and Q wave infarct patterns

*T*his chapter and the next examine one of the most important topics of clinical electrocardiography—the diagnosis of myocardial ischemia and infarction (ischemic heart disease). Basic terms are discussed first.

Myocardial Ischemia

Myocardial cells require oxygen and other nutrients to function. Oxygenated blood is supplied by the coronary arteries. If severe narrowing or complete blockage of a coronary artery causes the blood flow to become inadequate, ischemia of the heart muscle develops. *Ischemia* means literally to hold back blood.

Myocardial ischemia may occur transiently. For example, patients who experience angina pectoris with exercise are having transient myocardial ischemia. If the ischemia is more severe, necrosis of a portion of heart muscle may occur. *Myocardial infarction (MI)* refers to myocardial necrosis ("heart attack"), which is usually caused by severe ischemia.

This discussion focuses primarily on ischemia and infarction of the left ventricle, the predominant chamber of the heart. Right ventricular infarction is discussed only briefly.

Transmural and Subendocardial Ischemia

A cross-sectional diagram of the left ventricle is presented in Fig. 8.1. Notice that the left ventricle consists of an outer layer *(epicardium)* and an inner layer *(subendocardium)*. This distinction is important because myocardial ischemia may be limited to just the inner layer, or it may affect virtually the entire thickness of the ventricular wall (transmural ischemia).

Myocardial Blood Supply

Certain basic facts about the blood supply to the left ventricle are also important. The cardiac blood supply is delivered by the three main coronary arteries (Fig. 8.2). The right coronary artery supplies both the inferior (diaphragmatic) portion of the heart and the right ventricle. The left anterior descending coronary artery generally supplies the ventricular septum and a large part of the left ventricular free wall. The left circumflex coronary artery supplies the lateral wall of the left ventricle. This circulation pattern may be variable. Sometimes, for example, the circumflex artery also supplies the inferior portion of the left ventricle. MIs tend to be *localized* to

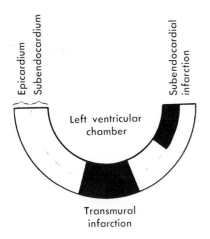

Fig. 8-1 Cross section of the left ventricle showing the difference between a *subendocardial* infarct, which involves the inner half of the ventricular wall, and a *transmural* infarct, which involves the full thickness (or almost the full thickness) of the wall. As discussed in the text, pathologic Q waves may be a marker of transmural infarction. However, not all transmural myocardial infarctions produce abnormal Q waves; in some cases, subendocardial (nontransmural) infarctions are associated with Q waves.

the portion (anterior or inferior) of the left ventricle supplied by one of these arteries.

Transmural Ischemia with Myocardial Infarction

The effect of a classic transmural MI on the ECG is examined in this chapter. Chapter 9 discusses the ECG patterns of subendocardial ischemia and non–Q wave infarction.

Transmural infarction is characterized by ischemia and ultimately necrosis of a portion of the entire thickness of the left ventricular wall. Not surprisingly, transmural infarction generally produces changes in both myocardial depolarization (QRS complex) and myocardial repolarization (ST-T complex).

The earliest ECG changes seen with an acute transmural infarction usually occur in the ST-T complex in two sequential phases. The *acute* phase is marked by the appearance of ST segment elevations and sometimes tall positive (hyperacute) T waves in certain leads. The *evolving* phase occurs hours or days later and is characterized by deep

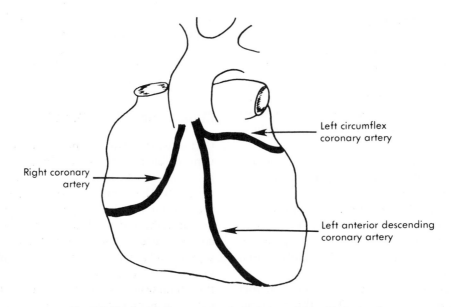

Fig. 8.2 The three major coronary arteries that supply blood to the heart.

T wave inversions in the leads that previously showed ST elevations.

Transmural MIs can also be described in terms of the location of the infarct. *Anterior* means that the infarct involves the anterior and/or lateral wall of the left ventricle, whereas *inferior* indicates involvement of the inferior (diaphragmatic) wall of the left ventricle (Fig. 8.3). The anatomic location of the infarct determines the leads in which the typical ECG patterns appear. For example, with an acute anterior wall MI, the ST segment elevations and tall hyperacute T waves appear in one or more of the anterior leads (chest leads V_1 to V_6 and extremity leads I and aV_L) (Fig. 8.4). With an inferior wall MI the ST segment elevations and tall hyperacute T waves are seen in inferior leads II, III, and aV_F (Fig. 8.5).

One of the most important characteristics of the ST-T changes seen with MI is their *reciprocity.* The anterior and inferior leads tend to show inverse patterns. Thus in an anterior infarction with ST segment elevations in leads V_1 to V_6, I, and aV_L, ST segment depression is often seen in leads II, III, and aV_F. Conversely, with an acute inferior wall infarction, leads II, III, and aV_F show ST segment elevation, with reciprocal ST depressions often seen in one or more of leads V_1 to V_3, I, and aV_L. (These reciprocal changes are illustrated in Figs. 8.4 and 8.5.)

The ST segment elevation seen with acute MI is called a *current of injury* and indicates that damage has occurred to the epicardial layer of the heart with a transmural infarction. The exact reasons acute MI produces ST segment elevation are complex and not fully understood. Normally the ST segment is isoelectric (neither positive nor negative) because no net current flow is occurring at this time. MI alters the electrical charge on the myocardial cell membranes. As a result, current flow becomes abnormal (current of injury) and produces ST segment deviations.

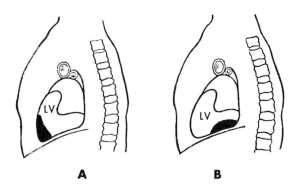

Fig. 8.3 Myocardial infarctions are generally localized to either the anterior portion of the left ventricle **(A)** or the inferior (diaphragmatic) portion of the walls of this chamber **(B).**

ECG Sequence with Anterior Wall Q Wave Infarction

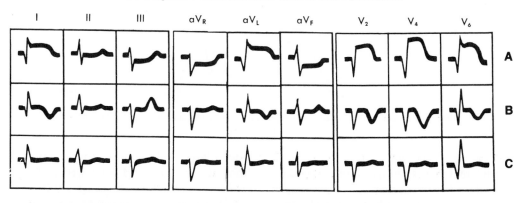

Fig. 8.4 A, Acute phase of an anterior wall infarction: ST elevations and new Q waves. **B,** Evolving phase: deep T wave inversions. **C,** Resolving phase: partial or complete regression of ST-T changes (and sometimes of Q waves). In **A** and **B,** notice the reciprocal ST-T changes in the inferior leads (II, III, and aV_F).

ECG Sequence with Inferior Wall Q Wave Infarction

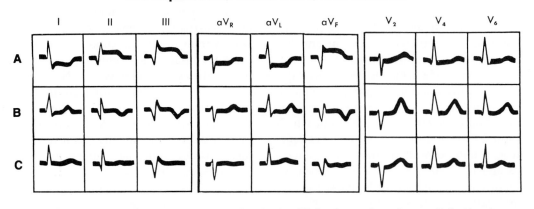

Fig. 8.5 A, Acute phase of an inferior wall myocardial infarction: ST elevations and new Q waves. **B,** Evolving phase: deep T wave inversions. **C,** Resolving phase: partial or complete regression of ST-T changes (and sometimes of Q waves). In **A** and **B,** notice the reciprocal ST-T changes in the anterior leads (I, aV$_L$, V$_2$, V$_4$).

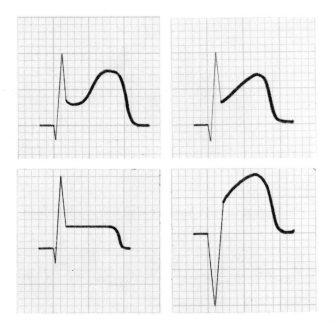

Fig. 8.6 Variable shapes of ST segment elevations seen with acute myocardial infarctions.

The ST segment elevation seen with acute MI may have different shapes and appearances (Fig. 8.6). Notice that the ST segment may be plateau shaped or dome shaped. Sometimes it is obliquely elevated.

The ST segment elevations (and reciprocal ST depressions) are the *earliest* ECG signs of infarction, and are generally seen within minutes of the infarct. Tall, positive (hyperacute) T waves may also be seen at this time (Figs. 8.7 and 8.8). These T waves have the same significance as the ST elevations. In some cases, hyperacute T waves actually precede the ST elevations.

After a variable time lag (hours to days) the elevated ST segments start to return to the base-

Fig. 8.7 Chest leads from a patient with acute anterior wall infarction. **A,** In the earliest phase of the infarction, tall, positive (hyperacute) T waves are seen in leads V_2 to V_5. **B,** Several hours later, marked ST segment elevation is present in the same leads (current of injury pattern), and abnormal Q waves are seen in leads in V_1 and V_2.

Fig. 8.8 Hyperacute T waves with anterior wall infarction. This patient was complaining of severe chest pain. Notice the very tall (hyperacute) T waves in the chest leads. In addition, slight ST segment elevations are present in lead aV_L and reciprocal ST depressions are seen in leads II, III, and aV_F. Notice the atrial premature beat (*APB*) in lead V_4.

line. At the same time the T waves become inverted in leads that previously showed ST segment elevations. This phase of T wave inversions is called the *evolving phase* of the infarction. Thus with an anterior wall infarction the T waves become inverted in one or more of the anterior leads (V_1 to V_6, I, aV_L). With an *inferior* wall infarction the T waves become inverted in one or more of the inferior leads (II, III, aV_F). (These T wave inversions are illustrated in Figs. 8.4 and 8.5.)

QRS CHANGES: Q WAVES OF INFARCTION

MI, particularly when transmural, often produces distinctive changes in the QRS (depolarization) complex. The characteristic depolarization sign is the appearance of new Q waves.

Why do certain MIs lead to Q waves? Recall that a Q wave is simply an initial negative deflection of the QRS complex. If the entire QRS complex is negative, it is called a *QS complex:*

A Q wave (negative deflection) in any lead indicates that the electrical voltages are directed away from that particular lead. With a transmural infarction, necrosis of heart muscle occurs in a localized area of the ventricle. As a result the electrical voltages produced by this portion of the myocardium disappear. Instead of positive (R) waves over the infarcted area, Q waves are recorded (either a QR or QS complex).*

In summary, abnormal Q waves are characteristic markers of infarction. They signify the loss of positive electrical voltages caused by the death of heart muscle.

The new Q waves of an MI generally appear within the first day or so of the infarct. With an anterior wall infarction these Q waves are

---

*As discussed in the next chapter, the question of pathologic Q waves with transmural necrosis is an oversimplification. Not all transmural infarcts lead to Q waves, and not all Q wave infarcts correlate with transmural necrosis.

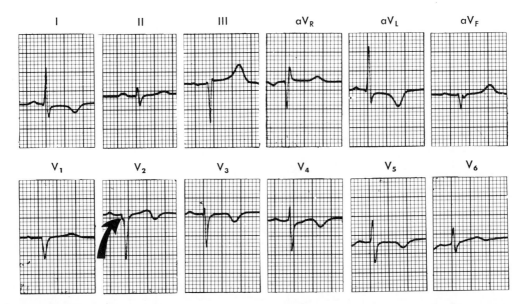

Fig. 8.9 Anterior wall infarction. The QS complexes in leads V_1 and V_2 indicate anteroseptal infarction. A characteristic notching of the QS complex, often seen with infarcts, is present in lead V_2 (*arrow*). In addition, the diffuse ischemic T wave inversions in leads I, aV_L, and V_2 to V_5 indicate generalized anterior wall ischemia or non–Q wave myocardial infarction.

seen in one or more of leads V_1 to V_6, I, and aV_L (see Fig. 8.4). With an inferior wall MI the new Q waves appear in leads II, III, and aV_F (see Fig. 8.5).

Localization of Infarctions

As mentioned, MIs are generally localized to a specific portion of the left ventricle, affecting either the anterior or the inferior wall. Anterior infarctions are sometimes designated as *anteroseptal, strictly anterior,* or *anterolateral/apical,* depending on the leads that show signs of the infarction (Figs. 8.9 to 8.11).

ANTERIOR WALL INFARCTIONS

The characteristic feature of an anterior infarct is *the loss of normal R wave progression in the chest leads.* Recall that normally the height of the R wave increases progressively as you move from lead V_1 to lead V_6. An anterior infarct interrupts this progression, and the result is pathologic Q waves in one or more of the chest leads.

Anteroseptal Infarcts

Remember from Chapter 4 that the ventricular septum is depolarized from left to right and that leads V_1 and V_2 show small positive (r) waves (septal r waves). Now consider the effect of damaging the

Fig. 8.10 Evolving anterior wall infarction. The patient sustained the infarct 1 week earlier. Notice the abnormal Q waves (leads I, aV_L and V_2 to V_5) with slight ST segment elevations and deep T wave inversions. Left axis deviation resulting from left anterior hemiblock is also present (see Chapter 7).

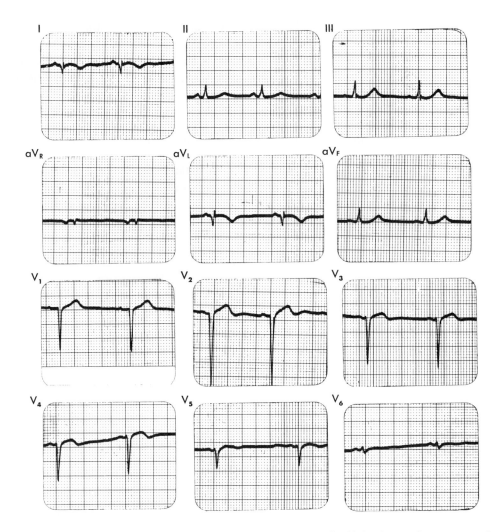

Fig. 8.11 Evolving anterior wall infarction. The infarct occurred 1 week earlier. Notice the poor R wave progression in leads V_1 to V_5 with Q waves in leads I and aV_L. The T waves are slightly inverted in these leads. In this ECG, right axis deviation is the result of loss of lateral wall forces, with Q waves seen in leads I and aV_L.

septum. Obviously, septal depolarization voltages are lost. Thus the r waves in leads V_1 and V_2 disappear and an entirely negative (QS) complex appears.

The septum is supplied with blood by the left anterior descending coronary artery. Septal infarction generally suggests this artery or one of its branches is occluded.

Strictly Anterior Infarcts

Normally leads V_3 and V_4 show RS- or Rs-type complexes. If an infarction occurs in the anterior

wall of the left ventricle, the positive R waves that reflect the voltages produced by this muscle area are lost. Instead, Q waves (as part of QS or QR complexes) are seen in leads V_3 and V_4. A strictly anterior infarct generally results from occlusion of the left anterior descending coronary artery.

Anterolateral or Anteroapical Infarcts

An infarction of the lateral or apical wall of the left ventricle produces changes in the more later-

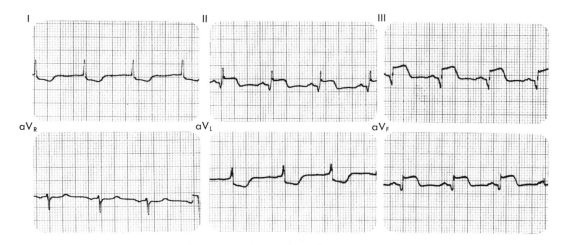

Fig. 8.12 Acute inferior wall infarction. Notice the ST elevations in leads II, III, and aV$_F$ and the reciprocal ST depressions in leads I and aV$_L$. Abnormal Q waves are also present in leads II, III, and aV$_F$.

ally situated chest leads (V$_5$ and V$_6$). With such infarctions, abnormal Q waves, as part of QS or QR complexes, appear in leads V$_5$ and V$_6$ (see Fig. 7.7). The infarcts are often caused by occlusion of the left circumflex coronary artery, but they may also result from occlusion of the left anterior descending coronary artery or even a branch of the right coronary artery.

Differentiating Anterior Wall Infarcts

The foregoing classification of anterior infarctions is not absolute, and infarct types often overlap. You can describe Q wave MIs by simply referring to any infarct that shows ECG changes in one or more of leads I, aV$_L$, and V$_1$ to V$_6$ as *anterior* and then specifying the leads that show Q waves and ST-T changes. Anterior infarctions associated with large Q waves in leads V$_1$ to V$_5$ or V$_6$ usually represent extensive damage and substantially reduced left ventricular function (ejection fraction) (see Fig. 8.11).

INFERIOR WALL INFARCTIONS

Infarction of the inferior (diaphragmatic) portion of the left ventricle is indicated by changes in leads II, III, and aV$_F$ (Figs. 8.12 to 8.14). These three leads, as shown in the diagram of the frontal plane axis, are oriented downward or inferiorly

(see Fig. 5.1). Thus they record voltages from the inferior portion of the ventricle. An inferior wall infarction may produce abnormal Q waves in leads II, III, and aV$_F$. This type of infarction is generally caused by occlusion of the right coronary artery. Less commonly it occurs because of a left circumflex coronary obstruction.

POSTERIOR INFARCTIONS

Infarctions can occur in the posterior (back) surface of the left ventricle. These infarctions may be difficult to diagnose because characteristic abnormal ST elevations may not appear in any of the 12 conventional leads. Instead, tall R waves and ST depressions may occur in leads V$_1$ and V$_2$ (reciprocal to the Q waves and ST segment elevations that would be recorded at the back of the heart). During the evolving phase of these infarctions, when deep T wave inversions appear in the posterior leads, the anterior chest leads show reciprocally tall positive T waves (Fig. 8.15).

In most cases of posterior MI the infarct extends either to the lateral wall of the left ventricle, producing characteristic changes in lead V$_6$, or to the inferior wall of that ventricle, producing characteristic changes in leads II, III, and aV$_F$ (Fig. 8.15). Because of the overlap between

Fig. 8.13 Inferior wall infarction. This patient sustained a myocardial infarction 1 month previously. Notice the abnormal Q waves and symmetric T wave inversions in leads II, III, and aV_F. In addition, T wave flattening is seen in lead V_6. After infarction, Q waves and ST-T changes may persist indefinitely or may resolve partially or completely.

inferior and *posterior* infarctions, the more general term *infero/posterior* can be used when the ECG shows changes consistent with either inferior or posterior infarction.

RIGHT VENTRICULAR INFARCTIONS

A related topic is right ventricular infarction. Clinical and autopsy studies have shown that patients with an inferoposterior infarct not uncommonly have associated right ventricular involvement. In one postmortem study, right ventricular infarction was found in about one of four cases of inferoposterior MI but not in cases of anterior MI. Clinically, patients with a right ventricular infarct may have elevated central ve-

nous pressure (distended neck veins) because of the abnormally high diastolic filling pressures in the right side of the heart. If the damage to the right ventricle is severe, hypotension and even cardiogenic shock may result. Atrioventricular conduction disturbances are not uncommon in this setting. The presence of jugular venous distension in patients with acute inferoposterior wall MIs should always suggest this diagnosis. Many of these patients also have ST elevations in leads reflecting the right ventricle, such as V_1 and V_{3R} to V_{5R}, as shown in Fig. 8.16 (see also Chapter 3).

Recognition of right ventricular infarction is of major clinical importance. Volume expansion

Fig. 8.14 Old inferior wall infarction. Notice the prominent Q waves in leads II, III, and aV_F from a patient who had a myocardial infarction 1 year perviously. The ST-T changes have essentially reverted to normal.

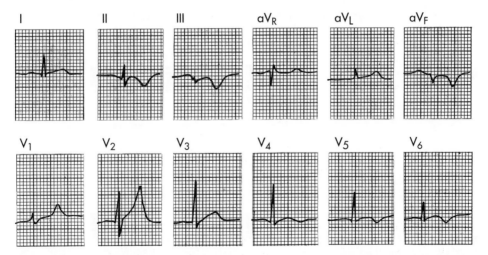

Fig. 8.15 Posterior infarction. Notice the tall R waves in leads V_1 and V_2. This patient had a previous inferior infarction (Q waves in leads II, III, aV_F) and probably a lateral infarction as well (T wave inversions in leads V_4 to V_6) Notice also the reciprocally tall, positive T waves in anterior precordial leads V_1 and V_2. (From Goldberger AL: *Myocardial infarction: electrocardiographic differential diagnosis,* ed 4, St Louis, 1991, Mosby.)

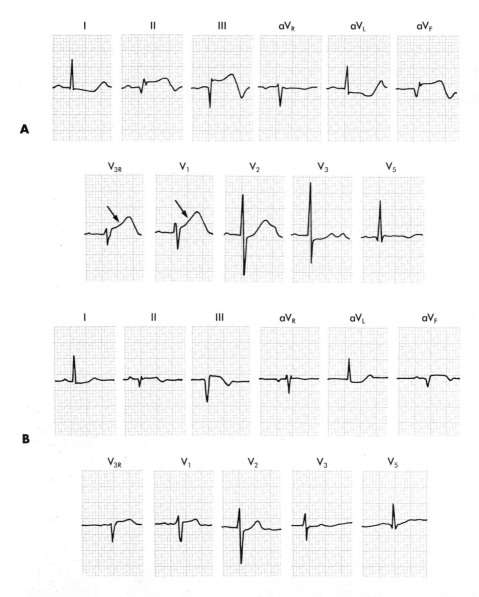

Fig. 8.16 Acute right ventricular ischemia with inferior wall infarction. **A,** Q waves and ST segment elevations in leads II, III, and aV$_F$ are accompanied by ST elevations *(arrows)* in the right precordial leads (V$_{3R}$ and V$_1$). The ST-T changes in lead V$_6$ are consistent with lateral wall ischemia. The ST depressions in leads I and aV$_L$ are probably reciprocal to inferior lead ST elevations. **B,** Follow-up tracing obtained the next day, showing diminution of the ST changes. (From Goldberger AL: *Myocardial infarction: electrocardiographic differential diagnosis,* ed 4, St Louis, 1991, Mosby.)

may be critical in improving cardiac output in patients who are hypotensive and have a low or normal pulmonary capillary wedge pressure despite elevated central venous pressure.

Sequence of Q Waves and ST-T Changes with Transmural Infarctions

To this point the ventricular depolarization (QRS complex) and repolarization (ST-T complex) changes produced by an acute MI have been discussed separately. As shown in Figs. 8.4 and 8.5, these changes occur sequentially.

Ordinarily, the earliest sign of transmural ischemia is ST segment elevations (with reciprocal ST depressions). The ST elevations (current of injury pattern) usually persist for hours to days. During this same period, Q waves begin to appear in the leads that show ST elevations. Once these changes have occurred, the ST segments start to return to the isoelectric baseline and the T waves become inverted during the evolving phase.

In the weeks or months after an infarct, what should you expect to happen to the Q waves and the ST-T changes just described? The answer is that you cannot make any certain predictions. In most cases the abnormal Q waves persist for months and even years after the acute infarction. Occasionally, however, the abnormal Q waves diminish in size and even disappear entirely. In some cases, abnormal T wave inversions persist indefinitely. In others, improvement occurs, but minor nonspecific ST-T abnormalities such as slight T wave flattening may persist (see Figs. 8.4 and 8.5).

Normal and Abnormal Q Waves

A frequently encountered diagnostic problem is deciding whether Q waves are abnormal. Not all Q waves are indicators of MI. For example, a Q wave is normally seen in lead aV_R. Furthermore, small "septal" q waves are normally seen in the left chest leads (V_4 to V_6) and in one or more of leads I, aV_L, II, III, and aV_F. Recall from Chapter 4 the significance of these septal q waves. The ventricular septum depolarizes

from left to right. Left chest leads record this spread of voltages toward the right as a small negative deflection (q wave) that is part of a qR complex in which the R wave represents the spread of left ventricular voltages toward the lead. When the electrical axis is horizontal, such qR complexes are seen in leads I and aV_L. When the electrical axis is vertical, qR complexes appear in leads II, III, and aV_F.

These normal septal q waves must be differentiated from the pathologic Q waves of infarction. Normal septal q waves are characteristically narrow and of low amplitude. As a rule, septal q waves are less than 0.04 second in duration. A Q wave is generally abnormal if its duration is 0.04 second or more in lead I, all three inferior leads (II, III, aV_F), or leads V_3 to V_6.

What if Q waves with a duration of 0.04 second or more are seen in leads V_1 and V_2? A large QS complex can be a normal variant in lead V_1 and rarely in leads V_1 and V_2. However, QS waves in these leads may be the only evidence of an anterior septal MI. An abnormal QS complex resulting from infarction sometimes shows a notch as it descends, or it may be slurred instead of descending and rising abruptly (see Fig. 8.9). Further criteria for differentiating normal from abnormal Q waves in these leads lie beyond the scope of this book.

What if a wide Q wave is seen in lead aV_L, or Q waves are present in leads III and aV_F? These waveforms can also occur normally. Although a discussion of the precise criteria for differentiating normal from abnormal Q waves in these leads is beyond the scope of this book, the following can be taken as general rules:

- An inferior wall MI should be diagnosed with certainty only when abnormal Q waves are seen in leads II, III, and aV_F. If prominent Q waves appear just in leads III and aV_F, the likelihood of MI is increased by the presence of abnormal ST-T changes in all three inferior extremity leads.
- An anterior wall MI should not be diagnosed from lead aV_L alone. Look for abnormal Q waves and ST-T changes in the other anterior leads (I and V_1 to V_6).

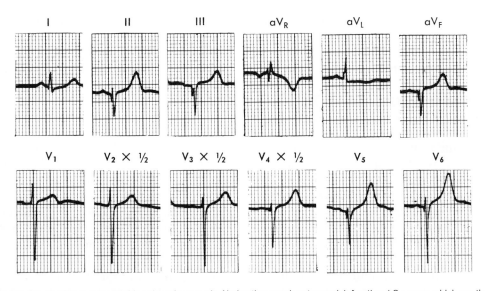

Fig. 8.17 Idiopathic hypertrophic subaortic stenosis. Notice the prominent pseudoinfarctional Q waves, which are the result of septal hypertrophy. (From Goldberger AL: *Myocardial infarction: electrocardiographic differential diagnosis*, ed 4, St Louis, 1991, Mosby.)

Furthermore, *just as not all Q waves are abnormal, all abnormal Q waves are not the result of MI*. For example, poor R wave progression in the chest leads, sometimes with actual QS complexes in the right to middle chest leads (e.g., V_1 to V_3), may occur with left bundle branch block (LBBB), left ventricular hypertrophy, and chronic lung disease in the absence of MI. Prominent noninfarctional Q waves are often a characteristic feature in the ECGs of patients with hypertrophic cardiomyopathy, including the subset of patients with classic idiopathic hypertrophic subaortic stenosis (Fig. 8.17). Noninfarctional Q waves also occur with dilated cardiomyopathy (see Fig. 10.18). As mentioned previously, the ECGs of normal people sometimes have a QS wave in lead V_1 and rarely in leads V_1 and V_2. Prominent Q waves in the absence of MI are sometimes referred to as a *pseudoinfarct pattern* (see Chapter 22).*

---

*For a more complete discussion of this subject, see Goldberger AL: *Myocardial infarction: electrocardiographic differential diagnosis*, ed 4, St Louis, 1991, Mosby.

Ventricular Aneurysm

After a large MI a ventricular aneurysm develops in some patients. An aneurysm is a severely scarred portion of infarcted ventricular myocardium that does not contract normally. Instead, during ventricular systole the aneurysmic portion bulges outward while the rest of the ventricle is contracting. Ventricular aneurysm may occur on the anterior or inferior surface of the heart.

The ECG may be helpful in making the diagnosis of ventricular aneurysm subsequent to an MI. Patients with ventricular aneurysm frequently have persistent ST segment elevations after an infarct. As mentioned earlier, the ST segment elevations seen with acute infarction generally resolve within several days. The persistence of ST segment elevations for several weeks or more is suggestive of a ventricular aneurysm (Fig. 8.18). However, the absence of persisting ST segment elevations does not rule out the possibility of an aneurysm.

Ventricular aneurysms are of clinical importance for several major reasons. They may lead

Fig. 8.18 Anterior wall aneurysm. The patient had a myocardial infarction several months before this ECG was taken. Notice the prominent Q waves in leads V₁ to V₃ and aV_L, the persistent ST elevations in these leads, and the reciprocal ST depressions in the inferior leads (II, III, and aV_F). The persistence of ST elevations more than 2 to 3 weeks after an infarction suggests the presence of a ventricular aneurysm.

to congestive heart failure. They may be associated with serious ventricular arrhythmias. A thrombus may form in an aneurysm and break off, resulting in a stroke or some other embolic complication.

Multiple Infarctions

Not infrequently, patients may have two or more MIs at different times. For example, a new anterior wall infarct may develop in a patient with a previous inferior wall infarction. In such cases

the ECG initially shows abnormal Q waves in leads II, III, and aV_F. During the anterior infarct, new Q waves and ST-T changes appear in the anterior leads. (The ECG of a patient with multiple infarcts [anterior and inferior] is presented in Fig. 8.19.)

Silent Myocardial Infarction

Most patients with an acute MI have symptoms. They may experience the classic syndrome of crushing substernal chest pain, or they may have

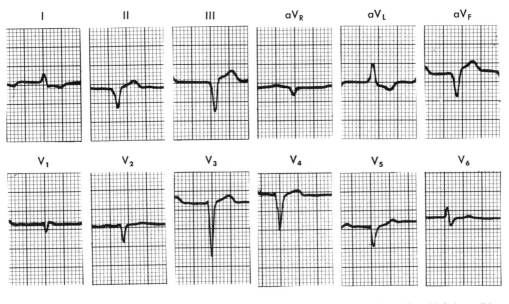

Fig. 8.19 Multiple myocardial infarctions. This ECG shows evidence of previous anterior wall and inferior wall infarcts. Notice the poor R wave progression and QS complexes in chest leads V_1 to V_5, as well as the QS waves in leads II, III, and aV_F.

atypical pain (e.g., a sensation like indigestion, upper back or jaw pain). Sometimes, however, patients may experience few if any symptoms ("silent" MI). Therefore it is not unusual for an ECG to show abnormal Q waves that indicate a previous infarction in a patient without a clinical history of definite MI.

Diagnosis of Myocardial Infarction in the Presence of Bundle Branch Block

The diagnosis of infarction is more difficult when the patient's baseline ECG shows a bundle branch block pattern or a bundle branch block develops as a complication of the MI. Then the ECG picture becomes more complex.

RIGHT BUNDLE BRANCH BLOCK WITH MYOCARDIAL INFARCTION

The diagnosis of an MI can be made relatively easily in the presence of right bundle branch block (RBBB). Remember that RBBB affects primarily the terminal phase of ventricular depolar-ization, producing a wide R' wave in the right chest leads and a wide S wave in the left chest leads. MI affects the initial phase of ventricular depolarization, producing abnormal Q waves. When RBBB and an infarct occur together, a combination of these patterns is seen: The QRS complex is abnormally wide (0.12 second or more) as a result of the bundle branch block, lead V_1 shows a terminal positive deflection, and lead V_6 shows a wide S wave. If the infarction is anterior, the ECG shows a loss of R wave progression with abnormal Q waves in the anterior leads and characteristic ST-T changes. If the infarction is inferior, pathologic Q waves and ST-T changes are seen in leads II, III, and aV_F. (An anterior wall infarction with the RBBB pattern is shown in Fig. 8.20.)

LEFT BUNDLE BRANCH BLOCK WITH MYOCARDIAL INFARCTION

The diagnosis of LBBB in the presence of MI is considerably more complicated and confusing than that of RBBB. The reason is that LBBB interrupts both the early and the late phases of

Fig. 8.20 Acute anterior wall infarction and the right bundle branch block (RBBB) pattern. The wide QRS complexes with an rSR′ wave in lead V_1, and a qRS pattern in lead V_5, indicate the presence of RBBB. A pattern of acute anterior wall infarction is indicated by the Q waves and ST elevations in leads I and aV_L and the marked reciprocal ST depressions in leads II, III, and aV_F. Finally, notice the left axis deviations caused by the left anterior hemiblock. This combination—left anterior hemiblock and RBBB—is an example of bifascicular block and may herald complete (trifascicular) heart block in patients with an acute anterior wall infarction (see Chapter 15).

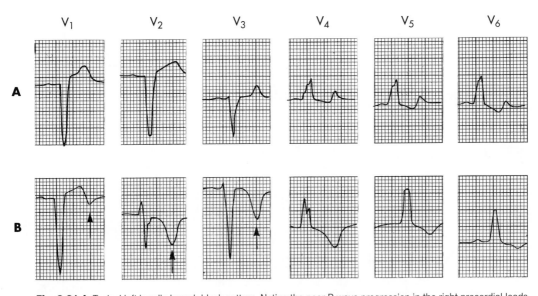

Fig. 8.21 A, Typical left bundle branch block pattern. Notice the poor R wave progression in the right precordial leads and the discordance of QRS and ST-T vectors reflected by the ST elevations in the right precordial leads and the ST depressions with T wave inversions in the left precordial leads. **B,** Subsequently the ECG from this patient showed the development of primary T wave inversions in leads V$_1$ to V$_3$ (*arrows*) caused by anterior ischemia and probable infarction. (From Goldberger AL: *Myocardial infarction: electrocardiographic differential diagnosis,* ed 4, St Louis, 1991, Mosby.)

ventricular stimulation (see Chapter 7). It also produces secondary ST-T changes. As a general rule, LBBB hides the diagnosis of an infarct. *Thus a patient with a chronic LBBB pattern who develops an acute MI may not show the characteristic changes of infarction described in this chapter.*

Occasionally, patients with LBBB manifest primary ST-T changes indicative of ischemia or actual infarction. The secondary T wave inversions of uncomplicated LBBB are seen in leads V$_4$ to V$_6$ (with prominent R waves). The appearance of T wave inversions in leads V$_1$ to V$_3$ (with prominent S waves) is a primary abnormality that cannot be ascribed to the bundle branch block itself (Fig. 8.21).

The problem of diagnosing infarction with LBBB is further complicated by the fact that the LBBB pattern has several features that resemble those seen with infarction. Thus an LBBB pattern can mimic an infarct pattern. As discussed in

Chapter 7, LBBB typically shows poor R wave progression in the chest leads because of the reversed way the ventricular septum is activated (i.e., from right to left, the opposite of what happens normally). Consequently, with LBBB a loss of the normal septal R waves is seen in the right chest leads. This loss of normal R wave progression simulates the pattern seen with an anterior wall infarct.

Fig. 7.5 shows an example of LBBB with poor R wave progression. In this case, anterior wall infarction was not present. Notice that the ST segment elevations in the right chest leads resemble the pattern seen during the hyperacute or acute phase of an infarction. ST segment elevation in the right chest leads is also commonly seen with LBBB in the absence of infarction.

As a general rule a patient with an LBBB pattern should not be diagnosed as having had an

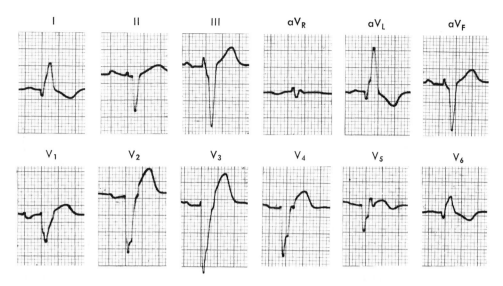

Fig. 8.22 Anterior wall infarction with left bundle branch block. Notice the prominent Q waves in the left chest leads as part of QR complexes (see text). (From Goldberger AL: *Myocardial infarction: electrocardiographic differential diagnosis*, ed 4, St Louis, 1991, Mosby.)

MI simply on the basis of poor R wave progression in the right chest leads or ST elevations in those leads. However, the presence of Q waves as part of QR complexes in the left chest leads (V_5 and V_6) with LBBB generally indicates an underlying MI (Fig. 8.22). In addition, the appearance of ST *elevations* in the left chest leads or in other leads with prominent R waves suggests ischemia (see Fig. 8.22, lead V_5), as do ST segment *depressions* in the right leads or other leads with an rS or a QS morphology. (The discussion of the ECG with ischemia and infarction continues in Chapter 9, which focuses on *subendocardial* ischemia and non–Q wave MI patterns.)

Review

Myocardial ischemia occurs when the blood supply to the myocardium is not adequate. *Myocardial infarction (MI)* refers to necrosis of the myocardium caused by severe ischemia.

Myocardial ischemia or infarction may affect the entire thickness of the ventricular muscle (*transmural* injury) or may be localized to the inner layer of the ventricle (*subendocardial* ischemia or infarction). Transmural MI often (but not always) produces a typical sequence of ST-T changes and abnormal Q waves. The ST-T changes can be divided into two phases:

1. The *acute* phase of transmural MI is marked by ST segment elevations (*current of injury* pattern) and sometimes tall positive T waves (hyperacute T waves).
2. The *evolving* phase is characterized by the appearance of deeply inverted T waves in leads that showed the hyperacute T waves and ST elevations.

These ST-T changes occur during a period of hours or days and usually resolve over weeks or months. During the first day or so after an MI, new abnormal Q waves may appear in one or more leads.

The persistence of ST segment elevations for more than 2 or 3 weeks after an acute MI may signify that a ventricular aneurysm has developed. The abnormal Q waves tend to persist but may become smaller with time and rarely may even disappear.

A Q wave MI can also be described in terms of its location. With an *anterior* infarction, ST segment elevations and abnormal Q waves occur in one or more of leads V_1 to V_6, I, and aV_L. Reciprocal ST depressions may be seen in leads II, III, and aV_F. With an *inferior* infarction, ST elevations and Q waves appear in leads II, III, and aV_F, and reciprocal ST depressions may be seen in one or more of the anterior leads.

Right ventricular MI is a common complication of inferoposterior infarcts. In acute cases the ECG may also show elevated ST segments in the right chest leads.

The pathologic Q waves of infarction must be distinguished from normal Q waves. For example, small normal "septal" q waves as part of qR complexes may be seen in the left chest leads (V_4 to V_6), in leads II, III, and aV_F (with a vertical electrical axis), and in leads I and aV_L (with a horizontal axis). These septal q waves are normally less than 0.04 second in width.

A QS wave may be seen normally in lead V_1 and occasionally in leads V_1 and V_2. Q waves may also be seen as normal variants in leads aV_F, III, and aV_L.

Multiple MIs can occur. In such cases the ECG shows old Q waves from the preceding infarct and new Q waves with ST-T changes from the current infarct.

When *right bundle branch block (RBBB)* complicates an acute MI, the diagnosis of both conditions is possible. The RBBB prolongs the QRS width, and lead V_1 shows a tall, positive final deflection. In addition, abnormal Q waves and ST segment elevations resulting from the acute MI are present in the chest leads with an anterior MI and in leads II, III, and aV_F with an inferior MI.

When *left bundle branch block (LBBB)* complicates an acute MI, the infarction may be difficult to diagnose because the LBBB may mask both the abnormal Q waves of the infarction and the ST segment elevations and T wave inversions of the ischemia. In addition, LBBB may produce QS waves in the right chest leads with ST segment elevations and poor R wave progression across the chest *without* MI. The presence of QR complexes in the left chest leads with LBBB is suggestive of underlying MI. Ischemia with underlying LBBB is suggested by the presence of T wave inversions in the right chest leads, ST segment elevations in the left chest leads (or in other leads with prominent R waves), or ST segment depression in the right precordial leads (or other leads with rS or QS waves).

Questions

See the end of Chapter 9.

9

Myocardial Ischemia and Infarction, Section II

Subendocardial ischemia and non–Q wave infarct patterns

*M*yocardial infarction (MI) may be associated with abnormal Q waves and the typical progression of ST-T changes described in Chapter 8. In other cases, however, myocardial ischemia (with or without actual infarction) may be limited to the *subendocardium* (inner layer) of the ventricle.

Subendocardial Ischemia

How can subendocardial ischemia occur without transmural ischemia or infarction? The subendocardium is particularly vulnerable to ischemia because it is most distant from the coronary blood supply and closest to the high pressure of the ventricular cavity. This inner layer of the ventricle can become ischemic while the outer layer (epicardium) remains normally perfused with blood.

The most common ECG change with subendocardial ischemia is ST segment depression (Fig. 9.1). The ST depression may be limited to the anterior leads (I, aV_L, and V_1 to V_6) or to the inferior leads (II, III, and aV_F), or it may be seen more diffusely in both groups of leads. As shown in Fig. 9.1, the ST depression with subendocardial ischemia has a characteristic squared-off shape. (ST segment elevation is usually seen in lead aV_R.)

Recall from the previous chapter that acute transmural ischemia produces ST segment elevation, a current of injury pattern. This results

from epicardial injury. With pure subendocardial ischemia, just the opposite occurs; that is, the ECG shows ST segment depression (except in lead aV_R, which often shows ST elevation).

In summary, myocardial ischemia involving primarily the subendocardium usually produces ST segment depression, whereas acute ischemia involving the epicardium usually produces ST elevation. (This difference in the direction of the injury current vector is depicted in Fig. 9.2.)

ECG CHANGES WITH ANGINA PECTORIS

The term *angina pectoris* refers to transient attacks of chest discomfort caused by myocardial ischemia. Angina is a symptom of coronary artery disease. The classic attack of angina is experienced as a dull, burning, or boring substernal pressure or heaviness. It is typically precipitated by exertion, stress, exposure to cold, and other factors, and it is relieved by rest and nitroglycerin.

Many (but not all) patients with classic angina have an ECG pattern of subendocardial ischemia, with ST depressions seen during an attack. When the pain disappears, the ST segments generally return to the baseline. (Fig. 9.3 shows ST depressions during a spontaneous episode of angina.)

The ECGs of some patients with angina do not show ST depressions during chest pain. Consequently, the presence of a normal ECG does not rule out underlying coronary artery disease. However, the appearance of transient ST depressions

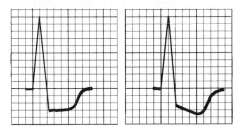

Fig. 9.1 Subendocardial ischemia may produce ST depressions.

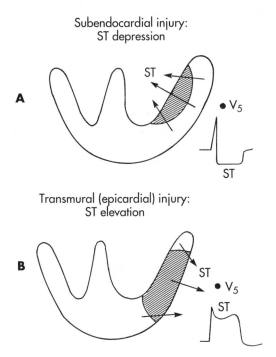

Fig. 9.2 A, With acute subendocardial ischemia the electrical forces *(arrows)* responsible for the ST segment are deviated toward the inner layer of the heart, causing ST depressions in lead V₅, which faces the outer surface of the heart. **B,** With acute transmural (epicardial) ischemia, electrical forces *(arrows)* responsible for the ST segment are deviated toward the outer layer of the heart, causing ST elevations in the overlying lead.

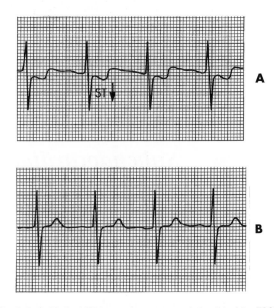

Fig. 9.3 A, Marked ST depressions are seen in lead V₄ of the ECG from a patient who complained of chest pain while being examined. **B,** Five minutes later, after the patient was given nitroglycerin, the ST segments have reverted to normal, with relief of angina.

in the ECG of a patient with chest pain is a very strong indicator of myocardial ischemia.

EXERCISE TESTING

Many patients with coronary artery disease have a normal ECG while at rest. During exercise, however, ischemic changes may appear because of the extra oxygen requirements imposed on the heart by exertion. To assist in diagnosing coronary artery disease, the cardiologist can record the ECG while the patient is being exercised under controlled conditions. *Stress electrocardiography* is usually performed while the patient walks on a treadmill or pedals a bicycle. The test is stopped when the patient develops angina, fatigue, or diagnostic ST changes or when the heart rate reaches 85% to 90% of a maximum predetermined rate predicted from the patient's age. This approach is known as *submaximal testing.*

Fig. 9.4, *A,* is the normal resting ECG of a patient, whereas Fig. 9.4, *B,* shows the marked ST depressions recorded while the patient was exercising. The appearance of ST segment depressions constitutes a positive (abnormal) result. Most cardiologists accept horizontal or downward ST depressions of at least 1 mm or more, lasting at least 0.08 second, as a positive (abnormal) test result (see Fig. 9.4, *B*). ST depressions of less than 1 mm (or depressions of only the J point) with a rapid upward sloping of the ST segment are considered a negative (normal) test response (Fig. 9.5).

Rest
Exercise

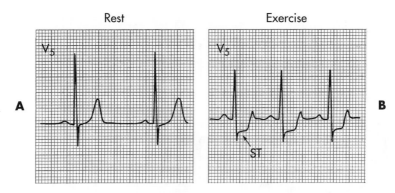

Fig. 9.4 A, Baseline rhythm strip from the positive exercise test of a patient with coronary artery disease. **B,** Notice the marked ST depressions with increased heart rate.

Lead V₅

Fig. 9.5 Lead V₅ shows physiologic ST segment depression that may occur with exercise. Notice the J junction depression *(arrow)* with sharply upsloping ST segments. (From Goldberger AL: *Myocardial infarction: electrocardiographic differential diagnosis*, ed 4, St Louis, 1991, Mosby.)

Exercise electrocardiography is often helpful in diagnosing coronary artery disease. However, like all tests, it may give both false-positive and false-negative results. For example, up to 10% of normal men and an even higher percentage of normal women may have false-positive exercise tests. False-positive tests (ST depressions without obstructive coronary disease) can also be seen in patients who are taking digitalis and in patients who have hypokalemia, left ventricular hypertrophy (LVH), ventricular conduction disturbances, or Wolff-Parkinson-White syndrome (see Chap-

ter 10). Furthermore, false-negative tests can occur despite the presence of significant underlying coronary artery disease. *Therefore a normal exercise test does not exclude coronary artery disease.**

In summary, subendocardial ischemia, such as occurs with typical angina pectoris (and as may sometimes be elicited with stress testing), often produces ST segment depressions in multiple leads.

---

*Consult the Bibliography for texts that discuss nuclear medicine imaging techniques with stress testing.

Fig. 9.6 Non–Q wave infarction in a patient who complained of severe chest pain. Subsequently, the patient's cardiac enzyme levels were elevated. Notice the marked, diffuse ST depressions in leads I, II, III, aV$_L$, aV$_F$, and V$_2$ to V$_6$, but the ST elevation in lead aV$_R$. These findings are consistent with severe subendocardial ischemia. Other unrelated abnormalities include a prolonged PR interval (0.28 second) and left atrial abnormality.

SILENT MYOCARDIAL ISCHEMIA

A patient with coronary artery disease may have episodes of myocardial ischemia *without* angina, hence the term *silent ischemia*. Silent ischemia is sometimes detected during exercise testing. Ambulatory ECG (Holter) monitoring is the most useful way of assessing silent myocardial ischemia (see Chapter 3). A 24-hour ECG monitoring of patients with coronary artery disease reveals a surprisingly high frequency of ST depressions *not* associated with angina. This important topic is discussed again later in this chapter.*

Subendocardial Infarction

If ischemia to the subendocardial region is severe enough, actual infarction may occur. In such cases the ECG may show persistent ST depres-

sions instead of the transient depressions seen with reversible subendocardial ischemia.

Fig. 9.6 shows an example of a non–Q wave infarction with persistent ST depressions. Is it possible for Q waves to appear with pure subendocardial infarction? The answer is that if only the inner half of the myocardium is infarcted, abnormal Q waves usually do not appear. Subendocardial infarction generally affects ventricular repolarization (ST-T complex) and not depolarization (QRS complex). However, as discussed at the end of this chapter, important exceptions may occur, and so-called *nontransmural* infarctions sometimes may be associated with Q waves.

Another ECG pattern sometimes seen in non–Q wave infarction is T wave inversions with or without ST segment depressions. Fig. 9.7 shows an infarction pattern with deep T wave inversions. (T wave inversions may also be seen in some cases of noninfarctional ischemia.)

In summary, non–Q wave infarction can be associated with either persistent ST depressions or T wave inversions.

*For additional information on this subject, see various texts cited in the Bibliography.

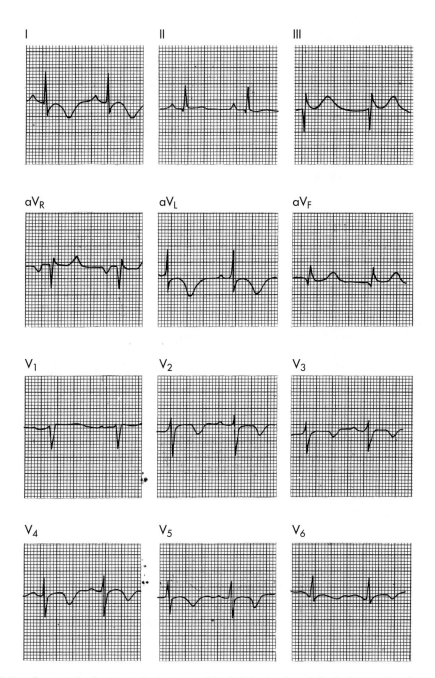

Fig. 9.7 Non–Q wave infarction in a patient who complained of chest pain and also had elevated cardiac enzyme levels. Notice the deep T wave inversions in leads I, aV$_L$, and V$_2$ to V$_6$. (Prominent Q waves in III and aV$_F$ represent an old inferior wall infarction.) Patients with acute myocardial infarction may have ST segment depressions or T wave inversions without Q waves.

Variety of ECG Changes Seen with Myocardial Ischemia

Myocardial ischemia clearly can produce a wide variety of ECG changes. For example, infarction may cause abnormal Q waves in association with ST segment elevations followed by T wave inversions. Ventricular aneurysm may be associated with persistent ST segment elevations. Subendocardial ischemia (e.g., during an anginal attack or a stress test) may produce transient ST depressions. In other cases, infarction may be associated with ST depressions or T wave inversions without Q waves.

ECG CHANGES ASSOCIATED WITH NONINFARCTIONAL ISCHEMIA

Myocardial ischemia does not always cause diagnostic ST-T changes. Several other patterns may be seen. In some patients the ECG may remain entirely normal during episodes of ischemia. In others the ST-T complex may display only subtle changes. For example, you may see just slight T wave flattening or minimal T wave inversions. These are *nonspecific ST-T changes* (see Chapter 10).

Nonspecific ST-T changes may be abnormal, but they are not definite indicators of ischemia. They may be a sign of ischemic heart disease, but they may also be caused by many other conditions, including drug effects, hyperventilation, and electrolyte abnormalities. Therefore you should *not* make a definite diagnosis of myocardial ischemia solely on the basis of nonspecific ST-T changes.

Prinzmetal's angina is another form of noninfarctional ischemia. Recall that the ECG with classic or typical angina often shows the pattern of subendocardial ischemia with ST segment depressions. However, an atypical form of angina (first reported by Dr. Myron Prinzmetal) is seen in a small but important group of patients. Their angina is atypical because during episodes of chest pain they have ST segment elevations, a pattern described previously with acute transmural MI. In Prinzmetal's angina the ST segment elevations are transient. After the episode of chest pain the ST segments usually return to the baseline, without the characteristic evolving pattern of Q waves and T wave inversions that occur with acute transmural MI. Thus Prinzmetal's angina is atypical be-

cause the ECG shows ST elevations rather than the ST depressions seen with typical angina.

Patients with Prinzmetal's angina are also atypical because their chest pain often occurs at rest or at night. (In contrast, patients with classic angina pectoris usually have chest pain with exertion or emotional stress.) Prinzmetal's angina pattern is significant because it is a marker of coronary artery *spasm* that causes transient transmural ischemia. These episodes of spasm may occur in patients with otherwise normal coronary arteries. In most cases, spasm is associated with high-grade coronary obstruction (Fig. 9.8). Increasing evidence implicates cocaine as another cause of coronary spasm.

At this point, the diverse ECG changes seen with ischemic heart disease can be summarized. These changes may include Q waves, ST segment elevations or depressions, tall positive T waves or deep T wave inversions, nonspecific ST-T changes, and even a normal ECG (Fig. 9.9).

Differential Diagnosis of ST Elevations and ST Depressions

ST segment elevations (current of injury pattern) are the earliest sign of acute transmural ischemia with infarction. Transient elevations are also seen with Prinzmetal's angina. ST segment elevations persisting for several weeks after an acute MI may be a sign of a ventricular aneurysm.

Not all ST segment elevations are indicators of ischemia. For example, *acute pericarditis* is associated with ST elevations (see Chapter 10). ST elevation may also occur as a *normal variant* (see Fig. 10.15). The ECGs of many young adults show ST elevations that are usually most prominent in the chest leads. This pattern of benign ST segment elevation is called the *early repolarization variant* (see Chapter 10). Finally, chronic ST elevations are often seen in leads V_1 and V_2 in association with the patterns of LVH or *left bundle branch block (LBBB)* (see Chapter 22).

Subendocardial ischemia is usually characterized by ST segment depression. However, not all ST depressions are indicative of subendocardial ischemia. For example, the ST-T changes associated with LVH (i.e., the "strain" pattern) were dis-

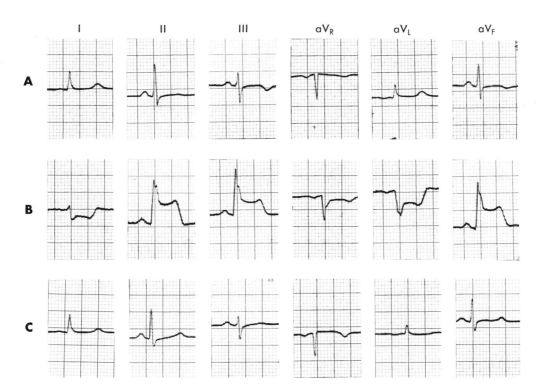

	I	II	III	aV_R	aV_L	aV_F

Fig. 9.8 Prinzmetal's (variant) angina with transient ST elevations in a 30-year-old man with a history of angina with exertion and at rest. **A,** The baseline resting ECG shows nonspecific inferior lead ST-T changes. **B,** With chest pain, marked ST segment elevations occur in leads II, III, and aV_F, and reciprocal ST depressions are seen in leads I and aV_L. The rightward axis shift and slight widening of the QRS complex are consistent with left posterior hemiblock. **C,** The ST segments return to baseline after the patient is given nitroglycerin. Cardiac catheterization showed severe right coronary obstruction with intermittent spasm producing total occlusion and transient ST elevations. (From Goldberger AL: *Myocardial infarction: electrocardiographic differential diagnosis,* ed 4, St Louis, 1991, Mosby.)

cussed in Chapter 6. As shown in Fig. 6.12, the ST segment may be slightly depressed with LVH. *Acute transmural ischemia* is another cause of ST segment depressions. Remember that acute anterior wall ischemia may be associated with reciprocal ST depressions in one or more of leads II, III, and aV_F. Conversely, acute inferior wall ischemia may be associated with reciprocal ST depressions in one or more of the anterior leads (I, aV_L, V_1 to V_3). Therefore whenever you see ST depressions, you need to look at all the leads and evaluate these changes in context.

The ST segment may also be depressed by two other important factors: the *digitalis effect* and *hypokalemia* (see Chapter 10). Digitalis may produce scooping of the ST-T complex with slight ST de-

pression (see Fig. 10.1). The ST segment may also be slightly depressed in the ECGs of patients with a low serum potassium level (see Fig. 10.8). Prominent U waves may also appear. In some cases it may be difficult to sort out which factors are responsible for the ST depressions you are seeing. For example, a patient with LVH may be taking digitalis and may also be having acute subendocardial ischemia.

Differential Diagnosis of Deep T Wave Inversions

Deep T wave inversions, as described previously, usually occur during the evolving phase of a Q wave MI (see Fig. 8.4, *B*) and also sometimes

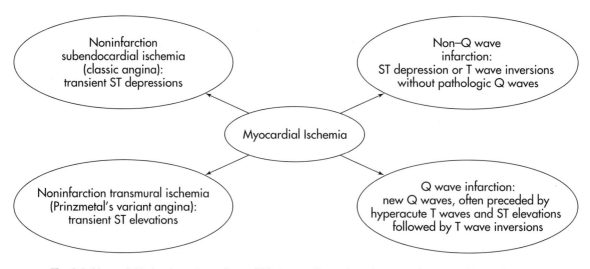

Fig. 9.9 Myocardial ischemia produces diverse ECG changes. T wave inversions may also occur with noninfarctional ischemia. Sometimes the ECG may be normal or show only nonspecific ST-T changes. (Adapted from Goldberger AL: *Myocardial infarction: electrocardiographic differential diagnosis,* ed 4, St Louis, 1991, Mosby.)

with a non–Q wave MI (see Fig. 9.7). These deep inversions are the result of a delay in regional repolarization produced by the ischemic injury.

However, just as not all ST segment elevations reflect ischemia, not all deep T wave inversions are abnormal. For example, T wave inversions may be seen normally in leads with a *negative QRS complex* (e.g., in lead aV_R). In adults the T wave may be normally inverted in lead V_1 and sometimes inverted in lead V_2. Furthermore, as mentioned in Chapter 4, some adults have a persistent *juvenile T wave inversion pattern,* with inverted T waves in the right and middle chest leads (typically V_1 to V_3).

In addition, not all abnormal T wave inversions are caused by MI. T wave inversions in the right chest leads may be caused by right ventricular "strain" (see Fig. 10.16) and in the left chest leads by left ventricular strain (see Fig. 6.10). Diffusely inverted T waves are seen during the evolving phase of pericarditis. Very deep, widely splayed T wave inversions (with a long QT interval and sometimes prominent U waves) have been described in some patients with cerebrovascular accident (CVA), particularly subarachnoid hemorrhage *(CVA T wave pattern)* (Fig. 9.10). The cause of these marked repolarization changes in some types of cerebrovascular injury is not certain, but they probably reflect changes in the autonomic nervous system. As described in Chapter 7, secondary T wave inversions (resulting from abnormal depolarization) are seen in the right chest leads with right bundle branch block (RBBB) and in the left chest leads with LBBB. Deep T wave inversions have also been reported after bouts of tachycardia (posttachycardia T wave syndrome) and after electronic ventricular pacing (postpacemaker T wave pattern). Patients with mitral valve prolapse syndrome may have slightly inverted T waves in the inferolateral leads (II, III, aV_F, V_5, and V_6).

This list of noninfarctional factors that cause T wave inversions is by no means complete. However, it should convey the point that *T wave inversions are not always indicative of myocardial ischemia* (see Chapter 22).*

---

*In some cases, deep diffuse *(global)* T wave inversions may occur without any identifiable cause. Also, see Chapter 22 for a more complete list of the differential diagnosis of the ST-T changes of MI.

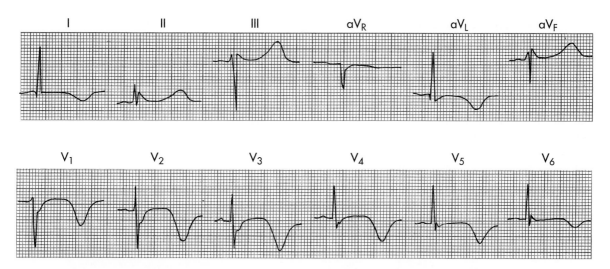

Fig. 9.10 The ECG of a patient with acute subarachnoid hemorrhage shows giant T wave inversions. Subarachnoid hemorrhage may cause deeply inverted T waves, usually with markedly prolonged QT intervals, simulating the pattern seen in myocardial infarction. (From Goldberger AL: *Myocardial infarction: electrocardiographic differential diagnosis*, ed 4, St Louis, 1991, Mosby.)

Complications of Myocardial Infarction

The major complications can be either mechanical or electrical. The *mechanical* complications include heart failure, cardiogenic shock, left ventricular aneurysm, rupture of the heart, pericarditis, papillary muscle dysfunction, infarct extension and expansion, and embolism. (The diagnosis of these problems is beyond the scope of this book.) The *electrical* complications include the arrhythmias and conduction disturbances that occur as a consequence of ischemia or infarction. MI can cause virtually any arrhythmia, including sustained ventricular tachycardia or ventricular fibrillation leading to cardiac arrest. (The general subject of arrhythmias is discussed in Part II.) The conduction disturbances include atrioventricular block (heart block) and intraventricular block (bundle branch block) (see Chapters 7 and 15).

ECG after Coronary Revascularization

ECG recognition of acute MIs (particularly with ST elevations or hyperacute T waves) is important

because such patients may be candidates for emergency coronary revascularization with catheterization and angioplasty-related procedures or with intravenous thrombolytic therapy. Acute revascularization therapies may alter the usual ECG evolution. Immediate successful revascularization very early after an acute MI may be marked by the return of elevated ST segments toward the baseline, without new Q waves. Deep T wave inversions may be seen in leads that showed ST elevations. However, Q waves often appear even after successful revascularization, although the intervention may lessen the amount of myocardium that is affected by the infarction. As a rule, the longer the time after the onset of ischemia or infarction, the less effect revascularization has on acute or evolving ECG changes.

The ECG in Myocardial Infarction: A Clinical Perspective

One final note of caution should be made. The ECG is a reasonably sensitive but hardly perfect indicator of acute MI. Most patients with an acute MI show the ECG changes described in Chapters 8 and 9. However, particularly during the early minutes or hours after an infarction, the ECG may be relatively nondiagnostic or even normal. Furthermore, an LBBB pattern may completely mask the changes of an acute infarct. Therefore the ECG must always be considered in clinical perspective, and the diagnosis of myocardial ischemia or infarction should not be dismissed simply because the ECG does not show the classic changes.

In addition, the traditional distinction between transmural and subendocardial (nontransmural) MIs on the basis of the ECG findings is an oversimplification. In some patients, extensive infarction may occur without Q waves; in others, nontransmural injury may occur with Q waves. Furthermore, current evidence suggests that subendocardial infarction may have as ominous a long-term prognosis as transmural infarction. For these reasons, electrocardiographers have largely abandoned the terms *transmural* and *subendocardial* and instead use *Q wave* and *non–Q wave* when describing an infarction.

Review

Subendocardial ischemia generally produces ST segment depressions, which may appear only in the anterior leads (I, aV$_L$, and V$_1$ to V$_6$), only in the inferior leads (II, III, and aV$_F$), or appear diffusely in both groups of leads. (Lead aV$_R$ usually shows ST segment elevations.)

These ischemic ST segment depressions may be seen during attacks of typical *angina pectoris*. Similar ST segment depressions may develop during exercise (with or without chest pain) in patients with ischemic heart disease. The presence of ischemic heart disease may be determined by recording the ECG during exercise *(stress electrocardiography)*. ST segment depression of 1 mm or more, lasting 0.08 second or more, is generally considered a *positive (abnormal)* response. However, *false-negative (normal)* results can occur in patients with ischemic heart disease and *false-positive* results can occur in normal people.

Ischemic ST segment changes may also be detected during ambulatory ECG (Holter) monitoring. Analysis of these records has shown that many episodes of myocardial ischemia are not associated with angina pectoris *(silent ischemia)*.

With *non–Q wave infarction* the ECG may show persistent ST segment depressions or T wave inversions. Abnormal Q waves do not usually occur with subendocardial infarction limited to the inner half of the ventricular wall.

With *Prinzmetal's angina,* transient ST segment elevations suggestive of epicardial or transmural ischemia occur during attacks of angina. Patients with Prinzmetal's angina often have atypical chest pain that occurs at rest or at night. In contrast, patients with classic angina, typically have exertional pain that is associated with ST segment depressions. Prinzmetal's (variant) angina pattern is generally a marker of coronary artery spasm with or without underlying coronary obstruction.

The ST segment elevations of acute transmural MI can be simulated by the ST elevations of Prinzmetal's angina, the normal variant ST elevations seen in some healthy people *(early repolarization pattern),* and the ST elevations of acute pericarditis (see Chapter 22).

The abnormal ST depressions of subendocardial ischemia may be simulated by the repolarization abnormalities of left ventricular hypertrophy, digitalis effect (see Chapter 10), or hypokalemia (see Chapter 10).

T wave inversions can be a sign of ischemia or infarction, but they may also occur in a variety of other settings (see Chapter 22), such as in normal variants or with ventricular hypertrophy, subarachnoid hemorrhage, and secondary ST-T changes from bundle branch block.

Questions—Chapters 8 and 9

1. Answer these questions about the ECG shown below:
   a. What is the approximate heart rate?
   b. Are ST segment elevations present?
   c. Are abnormal Q waves present?
   d. What is the diagnosis?

2. Answer these questions about the ECG shown below:
   a. What is the approximate mean QRS axis?
   b. Is the R wave progression in the chest leads normal?
   c. Are the T waves normal?
   d. What is the diagnosis?

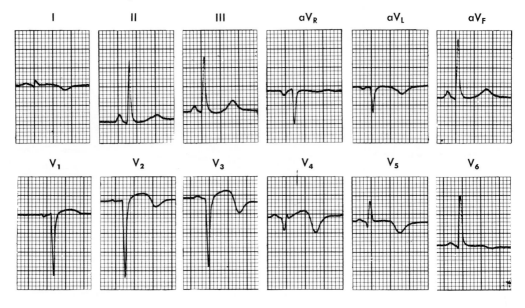

3. With acute transmural anterior wall ischemia, the ST segments in leads II, III, and aV_F are likely to be _____.

4. Persistent ST elevations several weeks or more after an infarction may be a sign of _____.

5. A patient with severe chest pain has persistent diffuse ST segment depressions with abnormal elevations of cardiac enzymes. Which of the listed conditions is the most likely diagnosis?
   a. Prinzmetal's angina
   b. Non–Q wave infarction
   c. Hyperacute infarction
   d. Angina pectoris

6. What ECG abnormality is shown, and what symptoms might this patient be having?

7. What conduction disturbance is present? What other major abnormality is present?

10

Miscellaneous ECG Patterns

*T*his chapter presents an electrocardiographic potpourri—brief discussions of a number of ECG patterns that have not been covered in detail to this point. Included are drug effects, electrolyte disturbances, systemic hypothermia, pericardial disease and myocarditis, early repolarization variant, pulmonary embolism, Wolff-Parkinson-White (WPW) preexcitation, and several other miscellaneous ECG patterns.

Drug Effects

Numerous drugs can affect the ECG. Generally the ECG changes are slight and nonspecific. However, distinctive changes can be produced by several commonly used drugs, including digitalis, quinidine and related agents, and the psychotropics.

Digitalis is used to treat heart failure and certain arrhythmias. One of its effects is to shorten repolarization time in the ventricles. This shortens the QT interval and is associated with a characteristic scooping of the ST-T complex *(digitalis effect)* as shown in Figs. 10.1 and 10.2. Notice that when digitalis effect occurs, the ST segment and T wave are fused together and it is impossible to tell where one ends and the other begins. Digitalis effect can be seen in patients taking therapeutic or toxic doses of any digitalis preparation (e.g., digoxin). Digitalis effect must be distinguished from *digitalis toxicity*, which refers to arrhythmias, conduction disturbances, and systemic side effects produced by excessive amounts of digitalis (see Chapter 16).

Quinidine, procainamide, and disopyramide are antiarrhythmic drugs with similar properties. In contrast to digitalis, they prolong ventricular repolarization. Therefore they may prolong the QT interval and flatten the T wave. In toxic doses

they may also prolong ventricular depolarization, leading to a widening of the QRS complexes.* Occasionally these agents produce prominent U waves resembling those seen with hypokalemia (discussed later in this chapter).

Quinidine and related drugs such as procainamide and disopyramide may in selected cases actually cause fainting or even sudden death due to torsade de pointes type of ventricular tachycardia (quinidine syncope), as described in Chapter 14. This *proarrhythmic* effect is most likely to occur with prolonged QT intervals and/or prominent U waves (Fig. 10.3).

Prolongation of the QT interval can occur with other cardiac antiarrhythmic drugs, notably sotalol and amiodarone. Psychotropic drugs (e.g., phenothiazines and tricyclic antidepressants) can markedly alter the ECG and in toxic doses can induce a fatal ventricular tachyarrhythmia or asystole. They may also prolong the QRS interval, causing a bundle branch block–like pattern, or they may lengthen repolarization (long Q-T-U intervals), predisposing patients to develop torsade de pointes. Fig. 10.4 presents the typical ECG findings of tricyclic antidepressant overdose, in this case in a young adult. Notice the prolonged QRS and QT intervals, as well as sinus tachycardia.

Electrolyte Disturbances

Abnormal serum concentrations of potassium and calcium can produce marked effects on the ECG. Hyperkalemia can, in fact, be lethal because of its cardiac toxicity.

---

*QRS prolongation may also occur with other antiarrhythmic drugs (e.g., propafenone, flecainide).

Digitalis Effect

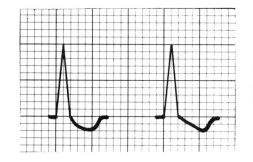

Fig. 10.1 Characteristic scooping of the ST-T complex produced by digitalis. (Not all patients taking digitalis exhibit these changes.)

Digitalis Effect

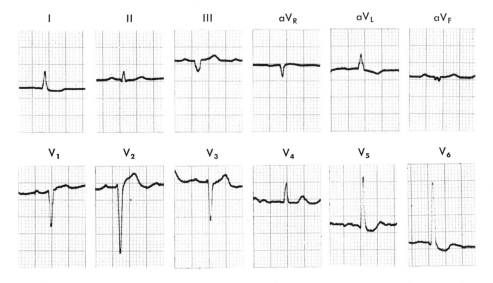

Fig. 10.2 The characteristic scooping of the ST-T complex produced by digitalis is best seen in leads V₅ and V₆. (Low voltage is also present, with a total QRS amplitude of 5 mm or less in all six extremity leads.)

Quinidine Effects and Early Toxicity

Fig. 10.3 Lead V₆ from the ECG of a patient with a quinidine blood level of 2.9 μg/ml (therapeutic range). Notice the prolonged repolarization with prominent U waves, similar to the pattern of hypokalemia. Patients in whom quinidine causes marked repolarization prolongation (often with large U waves) may be at increased risk for polymorphic ventricular tachycardia (torsade de pointes, see Chapter 14). This patient did, in fact, subsequently develop torsade de pointes.

Tricyclic Antidepressant Overdose

Fig. 10.4 **A,** This ECG from a patient with tricyclic antidepressant overdose shows three major findings: sinus tachy-cardia (from anticholinergic and adrenergic effects), prolongation of the QRS complex (from slowed ventricular con-duction), and prolongation of the QT interval (from delayed repolarization). **B,** A repeat ECG obtained 4 days later shows persistent sinus tachycardia but normalization of the QRS complex and QT interval.

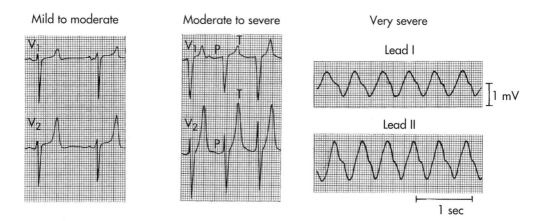

Fig. 10.5 The earliest change with hyperkalemia is peaking ("tenting") of the T waves. With progressive increases in the serum potassium concentration, the QRS complexes widen, the P waves decrease in amplitude and may disappear, and finally a sine-wave pattern leads to asystole unless emergency therapy is given.

HYPERKALEMIA

As shown in Fig. 10.5, progressive hyperkalemia produces a distinctive sequence of ECG changes affecting both depolarization (QRS complex) and repolarization (ST-T segments). The normal serum potassium concentration is between 3.5 and 5 mEq/L. The first change seen with abnormal elevation of the serum potassium concentration is narrowing and peaking of the T waves. As Fig. 10.5 demonstrates, the T waves with hyperkalemia have a characteristic "tented" or "pinched" shape, and they may become quite tall. With further elevation of the serum potassium concentration the PR intervals become prolonged and the P waves are smaller and may disappear entirely. Continued elevations produce an intraventricular conduction delay, with widening of the QRS complexes (see Figs. 10.5 and 10.6). As the serum potassium concentration rises further, the QRS complexes continue to widen, leading eventually to a large undulating (sine-wave) pattern and asystole.

Because hyperkalemia can be fatal, recognition of the earliest signs of T wave peaking may prove lifesaving. Hyperkalemia can be seen in several clinical settings. The most common is kidney failure, in which the excretion of potassium is reduced.

HYPOKALEMIA

Hypokalemia also produces distinctive changes in the ST-T complex. The most common pattern seen is ST depressions with prominent U waves and prolonged repolarization* (Figs. 10.7 and 10.8). With hypokalemia the U waves typically become enlarged and may even exceed the height of the T waves.

HYPERCALCEMIA AND HYPOCALCEMIA

Ventricular repolarization is shortened by hypercalcemia and lengthened by hypocalcemia (Fig. 10.9). In hypercalcemia the shortening of the QT interval is due to shortening of the ST segment. With marked hypercalcemia the T wave appears to take off right from the end of the QRS complex. High serum calcium concentrations may lead to coma and death. A short QT interval in a patient with mental status changes is sometimes the first clue to the diagnosis of hypercalcemia. Hypocalcemia lengthens or prolongs the QT interval, usually by "stretching out" the ST

---

*Technically the QT interval with hypokalemia may remain normal whereas repolarization is prolonged (as shown by the prominent U waves). Because the T waves and U waves often merge, the QT intervals cannot always be accurately measured.

Text continues on p. 121

Marked Hyperkalemia

Fig. 10.6 ECG of a patient with a serum potassium concentration of 8.5 mEq/L. Notice the absence of P waves and the presence of bizarre, wide QRS complexes.

Hypokalemia

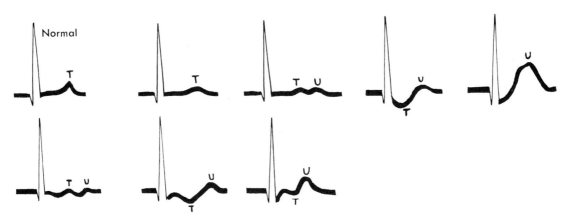

Fig. 10.7 The ECG patterns that may be seen with hypokalemia range from slight T wave flattening to the appearance of prominent U waves, sometimes with ST depressions or T wave inversions. These patterns are not directly related to the specific level of serum potassium.

Hypokalemia

Fig. 10.8 ECG leads from a patient with a serum potassium concentration of 2.2 mEq/L. Notice the prominent U waves, with flattened T waves.

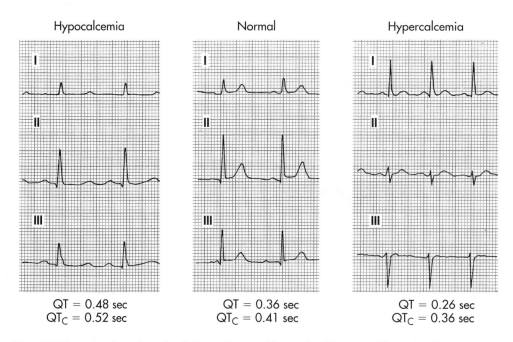

Hypocalcemia	Normal	Hypercalcemia

QT = 0.48 sec   QT = 0.36 sec   QT = 0.26 sec
QT_C = 0.52 sec QT_C = 0.41 sec QT_C = 0.36 sec

Fig. 10.9 Hypocalcemia prolongs the QT interval by stretching out the ST segment. Hypercalcemia decreases the QT interval by shortening the ST segment so that the T wave seems to take off directly from the end of the QRS complex.

Systemic Hypothermia

Fig. 10.10 Systemic hypothermia is associated with a distinctive bulging of the J point (the very beginning of the ST segment). The prominent J waves *(arrows)* with hypothermia are referred to as *Osborn waves.*

segment. Note, however, that patients may have clinically significant hypocalcemia or hypercalcemia without diagnostic ECG changes.

Hypothermia

Patients with systemic hypothermia may develop a distinctive ECG pattern in which a humplike elevation is usually localized to the junction of the end of the QRS complex and the beginning of the ST segment (J point) (Fig. 10.10). These pathologic J waves are sometimes called *Osborn waves.* This pattern disappears with rewarming.

Pericarditis and Pericardial Effusion

Pericarditis (inflammation of the pericardium) may be caused by a number of factors, including viral or bacterial infection, metastatic tumors, collagen vascular diseases, myocardial infarction (MI), cardiac surgery, and uremia.

As mentioned in Chapter 8, the ECG patterns of pericarditis resemble those seen with acute MI. The early phase of acute pericarditis is usually characterized by ST segment elevations. This is a current of injury pattern resulting from the inflammation of the heart's surface (epicardium)

that often accompanies pericardial inflammation. Fig. 10.11 shows an example of the ST segment elevations with acute pericarditis. A major difference between these elevations and the ones occurring with MI is their distribution. The ST segment elevations with acute MI are characteristically limited to the anterior or inferior leads because of the localized area of the infarct. The pericardium envelops the heart, and the ST-T changes occurring with pericarditis are therefore more generalized. ST elevations are typically seen in both anterior and inferior leads. For example, in Fig. 10.11 notice the elevations in leads I, II, aV_L, aV_F, and V_2 to V_6.

Not only does acute pericarditis affect ventricular repolarization (the ST segment), it also affects repolarization of the atria, which starts during the PR segment (the end of the P wave to the beginning of the QRS complex). In particular, pericardial inflammation often causes an atrial current of injury, reflected by elevation of the PR in lead aV_R and depression of the PR in other extremity leads and the left chest leads (V_5 and V_6). Thus with acute pericarditis the PR and ST segments typically point in opposite directions, with the PR being elevated (often by only 1 mm or so) in lead aV_R and the ST usually being slightly depressed in

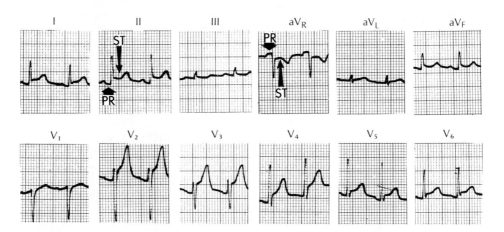

Fig. 10.11 Acute pericarditis causing diffuse ST segment elevations in leads I, II, aV_F, and V_2 to V_6, with reciprocal ST depressions in lead aV_R. By contrast, a concomitant atrial current of injury causes PR segment elevations in lead aV_R with reciprocal PR depressions in the left chest leads and lead II. (From Goldberger AL: *Myocardial infarction: electrocardiographic differential diagnosis,* ed 4, St Louis, 1991, Mosby.)

that lead. Other leads may show PR depression and ST elevation.*

Fig. 10.11 illustrates the subtle but often helpful repolarization changes seen with acute pericarditis. The presence of PR changes may be a useful clue in the differential diagnosis of ST segment elevation, suggesting acute pericarditis as the cause.

The ST elevations seen with acute pericarditis are sometimes followed (after a variable time) by T wave inversions (Fig. 10.12). This sequence of elevations and inversions is the same as that described for MI. In some cases the T wave inversions caused by pericarditis resolve completely with time and the ECG returns to normal. In other cases the T wave inversions persist for long periods.

The similarity between the ECG patterns of acute pericarditis and acute MI has been emphasized because both conditions may produce ST segment elevations followed by T wave inversions. As noted, however, the ST-T changes with

pericarditis tend to be more diffuse than the localized changes of MI. Another major difference is that pericarditis does not produce abnormal Q waves, such as those seen with certain infarcts. With MI, abnormal Q waves occur because of the death of heart muscle and the consequent loss of positive depolarization voltages (see Chapter 8). Pericarditis, on the other hand, generally causes only a superficial inflammation and does not produce actual myocardial necrosis. Thus abnormal Q waves never result from pericarditis alone.

Pericardial effusion refers to an abnormal accumulation of fluid in the pericardial sac. In most cases this fluid accumulates as the result of pericarditis. In some cases, however, such as myxedema (hypothyroidism) or rupture of the heart, pericardial effusion may occur in the absence of pericarditis. The major clinical significance of pericardial effusion is the danger of cardiac tamponade, in which the fluid actually "chokes off" the heart, leading to a drop in blood pressure and sometimes to cardiac arrest (see Chapter 17).

The most common ECG sign of pericardial effusion (with or without actual tamponade) is low

---

*This constitutes an exception to the earlier statement that repolarization of the atria generally is not apparent on the ECG (see Chapter 1).

Pericarditis: Evolving Pattern

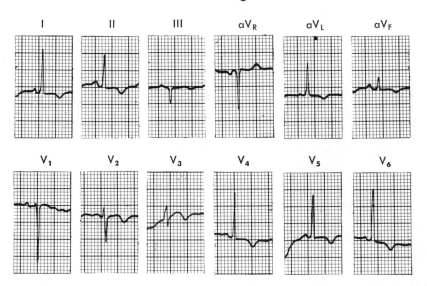

Fig. 10.12 Notice the diffuse T wave inversions in leads I, II, III, aV$_L$, aV$_F$, and V$_2$ to V$_6$.

voltage of the QRS complexes. In such cases the low voltage is probably due to short-circuiting of cardiac voltages by the fluid surrounding the heart.

The criteria for high voltage were mentioned in the discussion of hypertrophy patterns (see Chapter 6). *Low voltage* is said to be present when the total amplitude of the QRS complexes in each of the six extremity leads is 5 mm (0.5 mV) or less.* Fig. 10.2 shows an example of low voltage.

Following is a list of the major factors that can lead to low-voltage complexes (see Chapter 22).

• Obesity
• Emphysema
• Pericardial effusion
• Pleural effusion
• Diffuse myocardial injury (e.g., extensive MI or myocardial fibrosis)
• Hypothyroidism (myxedema)
• Infiltration of the heart muscle (e.g., amyloidosis)
• Normal variant

Obesity can cause low voltage because of the fat tissue that lies between the heart and the chest wall. Patients with emphysema have increased inflation of the lungs. This extra air acts to insulate the heart. Of the causes of low voltage listed, obesity and emphysema are among the most common. However, when you see low voltage (particularly with sinus tachycardia), you always need to consider pericardial effusion because it can lead to fatal tamponade (see Chapter 17).

As previously noted, myxedema (severe hypothyroidism) may cause pericardial effusion without actual pericarditis. Hypothyroidism also generally causes sinus bradycardia (see Chapter 11). Therefore the combination of low voltage and sinus bradycardia should suggest the possible diagnosis of myxedema.

Electrical alternans is another pattern that can occur with pericardial effusion and tamponade (Fig. 10.13). This pattern is characterized by a beat-to-beat shift in the QRS axis associated with mechanical swinging of the heart to-and-fro in a large accumulation of fluid. Electrical alternans is virtually pathognomonic of cardiac tamponade, although *not* every patient with tamponade manifests this pattern.

In summary, pericarditis causes a diffuse current of injury pattern with ST segment elevations in the anterior and inferior leads, followed by T wave inversions in those leads. Abnormal Q waves, however, are not seen with pericarditis alone. Pericardial effusion is one of the causes of low voltage on the ECG.

Myocarditis

A variety of conditions (e.g., certain viral infections) may be associated with inflammation of the heart muscle (myocarditis). The ECG findings with myocarditis are quite variable, ranging from nonspecific ST-T changes to the repolarization changes that occur with acute pericarditis. In some cases the ECG findings of severe myocarditis may exactly simulate those of acute MI, even with ST elevations initially and Q waves. Atrial or ventricular arrhythmias can occur with myocarditis, as can atrioventricular (AV) or ventricular conduction disturbances.

Early Repolarization Variant

Recall from Chapter 4 that the normal ST segment is isoelectric, riding along the baseline and gradually rising into the T wave (see Fig. 2.10). Although slight deviations (generally less than 1 mm) may be seen in the ECGs of normal people, more marked ST elevations may signify an abnormal condition (e.g., MI, Prinzmetal's angina, ventricular aneurysm, or pericarditis).

In Fig. 10.14 (the ECG of a *normal* young adult), notice the marked elevation of the ST segments. This is a benign variant known as the *early repolarization pattern.* With early repolarization the ST segments in the chest leads may rise to 3 mm above the baseline. Although most common in young people, these ST elevations can also occur in older persons, simulating the pattern seen with

---

*Low voltage in the extremity leads may or may not be accompanied by low voltage in the chest leads (defined as a total QRS amplitude of 10 mm or less in leads V_1 to V_6).

Electrical Alternans in Pericardial Tamponade

Fig. 10.13 Electrical alternans may develop in patients with pericardial effusion and cardiac tamponade. Notice the beat-to-beat alternation in the P-QRS-T axis; this is caused by the periodic swinging motion of the heart in a large pericardial effusion. Relatively low QRS voltage and sinus tachycardia are also present.

Early Repolarization

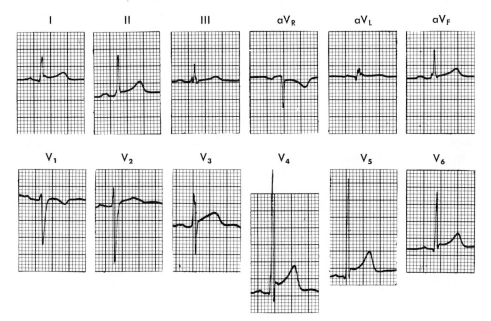

Fig. 10.14 ST segment elevation, usually most marked in the chest leads, is sometimes seen as a normal variant. This early repolarization pattern may be confused with the ST segment elevations of acute myocardial infarction or pericarditis.

acute pericarditis or MI. However, the elevations are stable and do not undergo the evolutionary sequence seen with acute pericarditis. Furthermore, they are not associated with reciprocal ST depressions (except in lead aV_R), contrary to what is often observed with acute MI.

Pulmonary Embolism

The ECG is *not* a sensitive test for pulmonary embolism. In some cases the obstruction produced by an embolus in the pulmonary artery system can lead to ECG changes, but generally no single pattern is always diagnostic. All of the following patterns may all be seen (Fig. 10.15):

- Sinus tachycardia (Arrhythmias such as ventricular ectopy and atrial fibrillation also occur.)
- A right ventricular "strain" pattern (inverted T waves in leads V_1 to V_4)
- The so-called $S_1Q_{III}T_{III}$ pattern, with an S wave in lead I and a new Q wave in lead III with T wave inversion in that lead (This pattern, which may simulate that produced by acute inferior wall MI, is probably due to acute right ventricular dilation.)
- Shifting of the QRS axis to the right

- ST segment depressions indicative of subendocardial ischemia
- An incomplete or complete right bundle branch block (RBBB) pattern (wide rSR' in lead V_1)

The appearance of these changes, particularly in combination, is suggestive but not diagnostic of pulmonary embolism. Many patients with massive pulmonary emboli have only minor, relatively nonspecific changes on their ECG. Thus both the diagnostic sensitivity and the specificity of the ECG with pulmonary embolism are limited. Figure 10.15 shows a classic example of the changes seen with pulmonary embolism.

Chronic Lung Disease (Emphysema)

Patients with chronic lung disease from emphysema often have a relatively characteristic combination of ECG findings (Fig. 10.16), including low voltage, poor R wave progression in the chest leads, and a vertical or rightward QRS axis in the frontal plane. Excessive pulmonary air trapping causes the low voltage. The poor R wave progression results, in part, from the downward displacement of the diaphragm. Thus the chest leads are actually placed *relatively* higher than usual. In

Acute Pulmonary Embolism

Fig. 10.15 Features occasionally seen with pulmonary embolism include sinus tachycardia, S waves in lead I with Q waves and T wave inversions in lead III ($S_1Q_{III}T_{III}$ pattern), and poor R wave progression with T wave inversions (right ventricular "strain") in chest leads V_1 to V_4 resulting from acute right ventricular overload.

Chronic Lung Disease

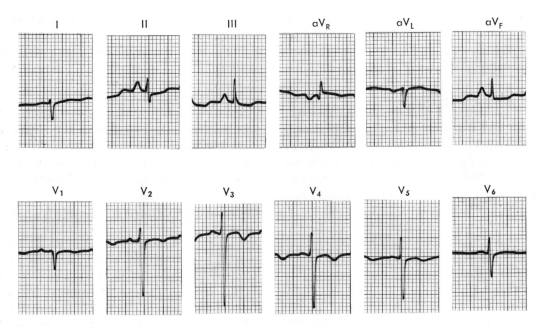

Fig. 10.16 Notice the characteristic relatively low voltages in the extremity leads, right axis deviation, P pulmonale, and poor R wave progression. The T wave inversions seen in leads V₁ to V₅ are due to right ventricular "strain." The P wave axis is also more vertical than usual (almost +90°).

addition, right ventricular dilation may contribute to the delayed chest lead transition zone. Finally, the anatomically vertical position of the heart in the chest of a patient with emphysema (and sometimes right ventricular enlargement) causes the mean QRS axis to be vertical or even rightward (greater than +100°). Tall, relatively narrow P waves caused by right atrial overload (see Fig. 10.16) may also be present, with a vertical or rightward P wave axis (+90° or so).

Congestive Heart Failure

Congestive heart failure (CHF) is a complex syndrome that may result from multiple causes, including ischemic heart disease, systemic hypertension, valvular heart disease, and cardiomyopathy. The ECG may provide helpful clues to a specific diagnosis in some of these patients. For example,

prominent Q waves and typical ST-T changes suggest underlying ischemic heart disease. Left ventricular hypertrophy patterns (see Chapter 6) may occur with hypertensive heart disease, aortic valve disease (stenosis or regurgitation), or mitral regurgitation. The combination of left atrial enlargement (or atrial fibrillation) and signs of right ventricular hypertrophy (RVH) should suggest mitral stenosis (see Fig. 19.1). Left bundle branch block (LBBB) (see Chapter 7) may occur with CHF caused by ischemic heart disease, valvular abnormalities, hypertension, or cardiomyopathy.

In some patients, marked enlargement and decreased function of the left (and often the right) ventricle occur without coronary artery disease, hypertension, or significant valvular lesions. In such cases the term *dilated (congestive) cardiomyopathy* is applied. Dilated cardiomyopathy can be idiopathic, or it can be associated with chronic ex-

ECG-CHF Triad

Fig. 10.17 Severe idiopathic dilated cardiomyopathy in a 29-year-old man. Poor precordial R wave progression simulates anterior wall infarction. The triad of relatively low QRS voltages in the extremity leads, prominent precordial QRS voltages, and poor R wave progression in the chest leads is highly suggestive of dilated cardiomyopathy. (From Goldberger AL: *Myocardial infarction: electrocardiographic differential diagnosis,* ed 4, St Louis, 1991, Mosby.)

cessive alcohol ingestion (alcoholic cardiomyopathy), viral infection, or some other etiology.

Patients with dilated cardiomyopathy from any cause may have a distinctive ECG pattern (the *ECG-CHF* triad), which is characterized by the following:

1. Relatively low voltages in the extremity leads, such that the QRS in each of the six extremity leads is 8 mm or less in amplitude
2. Relatively prominent QRS voltages in the chest leads, such that the sum of the S wave in either lead V_1 or lead V_2 plus the R wave in V_5 or V_6 is 35 mm or more.
3. Poor R wave progression defined by a QS- or rS-type complex in leads V_1 to V_4

When the ECG-CHF triad is present (Fig. 10.17), it strongly suggests underlying cardiomyopathy but does not indicate a specific etiology. The triad may occur not only with primary dilated cardiomyopathy but also with severe heart disease caused by previous infarction or significant valvular dysfunction. Furthermore, the ECG-CHF triad has only modest sensitivity; that is, its absence does not exclude underlying cardiomyopathy.

Wolff-Parkinson-White Pattern

The WPW syndrome is an unusual and distinctive ECG abnormality caused by *preexcitation* of the ventricles. Normally the electrical stimulus passes to the ventricles from the atria via the AV junction. The physiologic lag of conduction through the AV junction results in the normal PR interval of 0.12 to 0.2 second. Imagine the consequences of having an extra pathway between the atria and ventricles that would *bypass* the AV junction and *preexcite* the ventricles. This is exactly what occurs with the WPW syndrome: an *atrioventricular bypass tract** connects the atria and ventricles, circumventing the AV junction (Fig. 10.18).

Preexcitation of the ventricles with the WPW syndrome produces the following three characteristic changes on the ECG (Figs. 10-19 and 10-20):

1. The QRS is widened, giving the superficial appearance of a bundle branch block pattern. However, the wide QRS is caused not by a

---

*Formerly called the *bundle of Kent.*

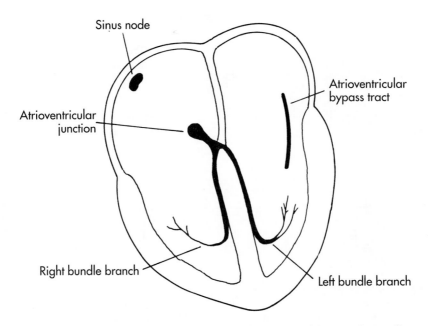

Fig. 10.18 Anatomy of the ECG pattern of the Wolff-Parkinson-White preexcitation pattern. In a small percentage of people an accessory fiber (atrioventricular bypass tract) connects the atria and ventricles. (The consequences of this extra conduction path are discussed in the text.)

Wolff-Parkinson-White Preexcitation

- Short PR
- Wide QRS
- Delta Wave (arrow)

Fig. 10.19 Preexcitation via the bypass tract in the Wolff-Parkinson-White (WPW) pattern is associated with a triad of findings.

delay in ventricular depolarization but by early stimulation of the ventricles. (The QRS is widened to the degree that the PR is shortened.)
2. The PR is shortened (often but not always to less than 0.12 second) because of ventricular preexcitation.
3. The upstroke of the QRS complex is slurred or notched. This is called a *delta* wave.

Figs. 10.19 and 10.20 show the WPW pattern, with its classic triad of a widened QRS, a short PR interval, and a delta wave. Notice that the pattern superficially resembles a bundle branch block pattern because of the widened QRS complexes. Depending on which area of the ventricles is preexcited first, the ECG may show a pattern simulating that of either RBBB with tall R waves in the right chest leads or LBBB with a predominantly negative QS in lead V_1.

The significance of WPW preexcitation is twofold:
1. Patients with this pattern are prone to arrhythmias, especially paroxysmal supraventricular tachycardia (PSVT) (Fig. 10.21).
2. The ECG of these patients is often mistaken as indicating a bundle branch block or MI (see Fig. 10.20).

The WPW syndrome predisposes patients to develop paroxysmal supraventricular tachycardia (PSVT) because of the presence of an extra conduction pathway. For example, a premature im-

Fig. 10.20 Notice the characteristic triad of the Wolff-Parkinson-White pattern: wide QRS complexes, short PR intervals, and delta waves *(arrows)* that are negative in some leads (e.g., II, III, and aV$_F$) and positive in others (aV$_L$ and V$_4$ to V$_6$). The Q waves in leads II, III, and aV$_F$ are the result of abnormal ventricular conduction (negative delta waves) rather than an inferior myocardial infarction.

pulse traveling down the AV junction may recycle up the accessory pathway and then back down the AV junction, and so on.* This type of recirculating impulse is an example of *reentry*.

Another type of preexcitation variant, the Lown-Ganong-Levine (LGL) syndrome, is caused by a bypass tract that connects the atria and AV junction. Bypassing the AV node results in a short PR interval (less than 0.12 second). However, the QRS width is not prolonged, because ventricular activation occurs normally. Therefore the LGL pattern consists of a normal-width QRS complex with a short PR interval and no delta wave; the WPW consists of a wide QRS complex with a short PR interval and a delta wave (see Fig. 10.19).

Patients with the LGL pattern may also have reentrant-type PSVT or paroxysmal atrial fibrillation or flutter.*

Differential Diagnosis of Wide QRS Complexes

The major ECG patterns that produce a widened QRS complex can be divided into four major categories (also see Chapter 22):
1. Bundle branch blocks, including the classic RBBB and LBBB patterns
2. "Toxic" conduction delays caused by some extrinsic factor, such as hyperkalemia or drugs

---

*When PSVT develops in a patient with the WPW syndrome, the QRS complex generally becomes narrow. The widened QRS seen with WPW syndrome during normal sinus rhythm occurs because the stimulus travels concomitantly down the bypass tract and down the AV junction, resulting in a *fusion* beat. When PSVT occurs, the impulse usually travels down the AV junction and back up the bypass tract in a retrograde fashion, resulting in a loss of the delta wave. (The role of bypass tracts in PSVT is discussed further in Chapters 12 and 18.)

---

*Most people with a short PR interval and normal QRS do not have LGL preexcitation, however. A relatively short PR interval may be seen as a normal variant, without a bypass tract, because of accelerated AV conduction. Therefore you should not "overread" an ECG on which the only noteworthy finding is a short PR interval.

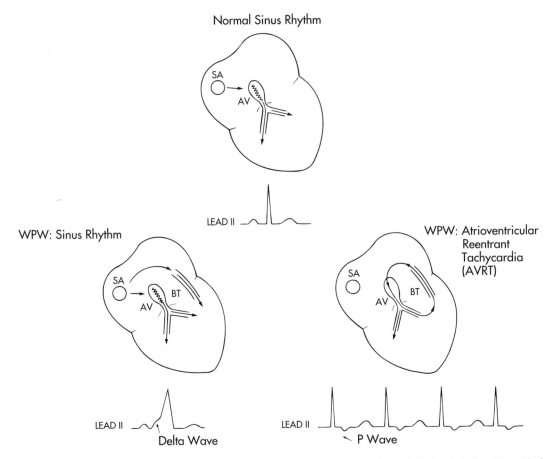

Fig. 10.21 Conduction during sinus rhythm in the normal heart *(top)* spreads from the sinoatrial *(SA)* node to the atrioventricular *(AV)* node and then down the bundle branches. The jagged line indicates physiologic slowing of conduction in the AV node. With Wolff-Parkinson-White *(WPW)* syndrome *(bottom left)*, an abnormal accessory conduction pathway called a bypass tract *(BT)* connects the atria and ventricles. With WPW, during sinus rhythm the electrical impulse is conducted quickly down the bypass tract, preexciting the ventricles before the impulse arrives via the AV node. Consequently, the PR interval is short and the QRS complex is wide, with slurring at its onset *(delta wave)*. WPW predisposes patients to develop an atrioventricular reentrant tachycardia (AVRT) *(bottom right)* in which a premature atrial beat may spread down the normal pathway to the ventricles, travel back up the bypass tract, and recirculate down the AV node again. This reentrant loop can repeat itself over and over, resulting in a tachycardia. Notice the normal QRS complex and often negative P wave in lead II during this type of bypass-tract tachycardia (see Chapter 12).

(e.g., quinidine, propafenone, flecainide and other related antiarrhythmics, phenothiazines, and tricyclic antidepressants)

3. Beats arising in the ventricles, which may be ventricular premature beats (see Chapter 14), ventricular escape beats (see Fig. 17.14), or pacemaker beats (see Chapter 7)

4. WPW-type preexcitation

Differentiation among these possibilities is usually easy. The ECG effects of RBBB and LBBB have already been described (see Chapter 7). Hyperkalemia produces widening of the QRS complex, often with loss of P waves. Widening of the QRS complex in any patient who is taking an antiarrhythmic or a psychotropic agent should always suggest possible drug toxicity. Pacemak-

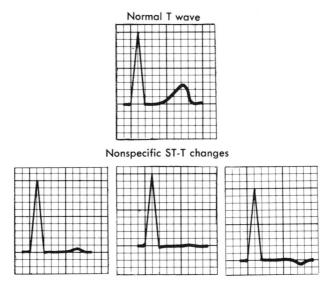

Fig. 10.22 Flattening of the T wave (*bottom left* and *middle*) and slight T wave inversion *(bottom right)* are abnormal but relatively nonspecific ECG changes that may be caused by numerous factors.

ers generally produce an LBBB pattern with a pacemaker spike before each QRS complex. The WPW pattern is recognized by the combination of a short PR interval, a wide QRS complex, and a delta wave.

ST-T Changes: Specific and Nonspecific

The concluding topic of Part 1 is a review of the major factors that cause ST-T (repolarization) changes. The term *nonspecific ST-T change* (defined in Chapter 9) is commonly used in clinical electrocardiography. Many factors (e.g., drugs, ischemia, electrolyte imbalances, infections, and pulmonary disease) can affect the ECG. As already mentioned, the repolarization phase (ST-T complex) is particularly sensitive to such effects and can show a variety of nonspecific changes as a result of multiple factors (Figs. 10.22 and 10.23). These changes include slight ST depressions, T wave flattening, and slight T wave inversions (see Fig. 10-22).

In contrast to these nonspecific ST-T changes, certain fairly specific changes are associated with particular conditions (e.g., the tall, tented T waves

of hyperkalemia). Some of these relatively specific ST-T changes are shown in Fig. 10.24. However, even such apparently specific changes can be misleading. For example, ST elevations are characteristic of acute transmural ischemia, but they are also seen in ventricular aneurysms, pericarditis, and benign (normal) early repolarization. Similarly, deep T wave inversions are most characteristic of ischemia but may occur in other conditions as well (see Chapters 9 and 22).

In summary, repolarization abnormalities can be grouped into two general categories. *Nonspecific* ST-T changes include slight ST segment deviation and flattening or inversion of the T wave. These changes are not diagnostic of any particular condition but must always be interpreted in clinical context. The relatively *specific* ST-T changes are more strongly but not always definitively diagnostic of some particular underlying cause (e.g., hyperkalemia or myocardial ischemia).

Pediatric Electrocardiography

The normal ECG patterns seen in children differ considerably from those in adults (see Chapter 4).

Fig. 10.23 ECG showing nonspecific ST-T changes. Notice the diffuse T wave flattening.

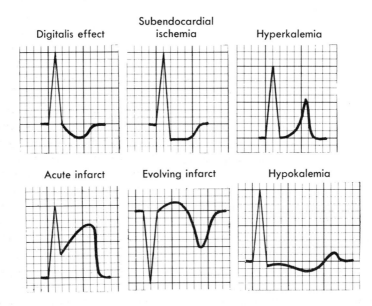

Fig. 10.24 Examples of relatively specific ST-T changes. Note, however, that the changes are not absolutely specific for the abnormalities shown.

Fig. 10.25 The ECG of this healthy neonate shows a pattern resembling that of right ventricular hypertrophy, with tall right precordial R waves and right axis deviation. This pattern reflects the physiologic predominance of the right ventricle during fetal development. Notice also the sinus tachycardia and relatively narrow QRS complexes.

The topic of pediatric electrocardiography falls outside the scope of this book, but a few critical points of difference between pediatric and adult ECGs are mentioned briefly. The normal ECG of a neonate resembles the pattern seen in RVH, with tall R waves in the right chest leads and right axis deviation (Fig. 10.25). During the first decade of life the T waves in the right to middle chest leads are normally inverted. This pattern, which sometimes persists into adolescence and adulthood, is called the *juvenile T wave variant*. Children and young adults may also have high voltage in the chest leads as a normal variant (see Chapter 6).

Review

The ECG can be influenced by numerous factors, including many *drugs*. *Digitalis effect* refers to the characteristic scooped-out depression of the ST segment produced by therapeutic doses of digitalis. (*Digitalis toxicity* refers to the arrhythmias and conduction disturbances produced by excessive doses of digitalis.) *Quinidine, procainamide, disopyramide,* and certain *psychotropic drugs* can prolong the QT interval and in toxic doses can markedly widen the QRS complex. These drugs, as well as *sotalol,* may also cause a potentially lethal type of ventricular tachycardia called *torsade de pointes* (see Chapter 14). Patients likely to develop this complication usually show prolonged QT intervals and/or large U waves. *Amiodarone* is a drug that typically prolongs the QT interval, even at therapeutic doses.

    Electrolyte disturbances can also affect the ECG:

1. *Hyperkalemia* typically produces a sequence of changes. First the T wave narrows and peaks ("tents"). Further elevation of the serum potassium concentration leads to

prolongation of the PR interval and then to loss of P waves and widening of the QRS complex, followed by a sine-wave pattern and asystole.

2. *Hypokalemia* may produce ST depressions and prominent U waves. The QT interval becomes prolonged. (In some cases you are actually measuring the QU interval, and not the QT interval, because it may be impossible to tell where the T wave ends and the U wave begins.)

3. *Hypercalcemia* may shorten the QT interval, and *hypocalcemia* may prolong it.

With *systemic hypothermia* the ECG shows a humplike elevation located at the junction (J point) of the end of the QRS complex and the beginning of the ST segment. The pattern disappears with rewarming.

Pericarditis produces diffuse ST segment elevations, usually in one or more of the chest leads and also in leads I, aV_L, II, and aV_F. PR segment elevation in lead aV_R with PR depression in other leads may be caused by an atrial current of injury. Abnormal Q waves do not develop. After a variable period the ST segment elevations may be followed by T wave inversions.

Pericardial effusion often produces *low voltage* of the QRS complex (amplitude of 5 mm or less in all six extremity leads). Low voltage is not specific for pericardial effusion because it may also occur with obesity, emphysema, and diffuse myocardial injury or infiltration. In addition, low voltage may occur as a normal variant.

Pericardial effusion complicated by *cardiac tamponade* is usually associated with sinus tachycardia and low voltage complexes. Some of these patients also have *electrical alternans*, a pattern characterized by a beat-to-beat shift in the QRS axis.

Myocarditis can produce ST-T changes that are nonspecific or that resemble the changes of pericarditis or myocardial infarction (MI). It may also be associated with arrhythmias.

Normally the ST segment is isoelectric. However, the ECGs of some healthy people, particularly young men, may show normal ST segment elevations *(early repolarization variant)*, usually best seen in the chest leads (up to 3 mm of elevation). The pattern may simulate that of acute MI or pericarditis, but it does not show the successive changes that usually occur with those pathologies.

Pulmonary embolism may produce any of the following patterns:

1. Sinus tachycardia and various arrhythmias
2. Right ventricular strain T wave inversions
3. $S_I Q_{III} T_{III}$
4. Right axis shift
5. ST depressions resulting from subendocardial ischemia
6. Acute right bundle branch block

The *Wolff-Parkinson-White (WPW) pattern* shows the following:

1. A short PR interval (usually but not always less than 0.12 second)
2. A wide QRS complex
3. Slurring or notching of the initial part of the QRS complex (termed a *delta* wave)

Patients with the WPW pattern are particularly prone to attacks of reentrant-type paroxysmal supraventricular tachycardia. Another form of preexcitation, the *Lown-Ganong-Levine syndrome*, is characterized by a short PR interval and a normal QRS complex.

The differential diagnosis of ECG patterns with a wide QRS complex includes four major possibilities:

1. Right or left bundle branch block
2. Toxic conduction delays caused by hyperkalemia or certain drugs
3. Beats arising in the ventricles, such as ventricular premature beats or pacemaker beats
4. WPW preexcitation

Questions

1. Which of the following factors can produce ST segment elevations?
   a. Hypokalemia
   b. Early repolarization pattern
   c. Digitalis effect
   d. Ventricular aneurysm
   e. Hypocalcemia
   f. Right bundle branch block
   g. Pericarditis
2. Match ECGs *A, B,* and *C* with the following causes:
   a. Digitalis effect
   b. Hyperkalemia
   c. Hypokalemia

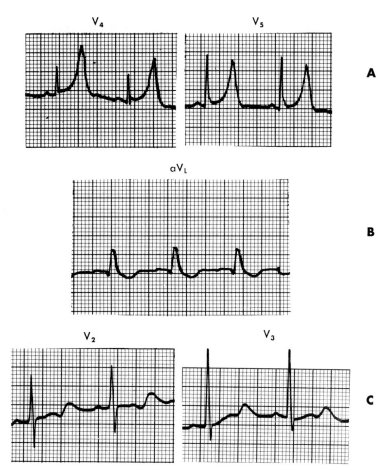

3. What caused the wide QRS complex in the ECG shown below?
   a. Right bundle branch block
   b. Quinidine toxicity
   c. Posterolateral infarction
   d. Wolff-Parkinson-White pattern
   e. Hyperkalemia

Part Two

Cardiac Rhythm Disturbances

Sinus Rhythms

Normal Sinus Rhythm

The diagnosis of normal sinus rhythm was described in Chapter 3. When the sinus (or sinoatrial [SA] node) is pacing the heart, atrial depolarization spreads from right to left and downward toward the atrioventricular (AV) junction. An arrow representing this depolarization wave points downward and toward the left. Therefore with normal sinus rhythm the P wave is negative in lead aV_R and positive in lead II (see Figs. 4.3 and 11.1).

By convention, *normal sinus rhythm* is usually defined as sinus rhythm with a heart rate between 60 and 100 beats/min. Sinus rhythm with a heart rate of less than 60 beats/min is called *sinus bradycardia.** Sinus rhythm with a heart rate greater than 100 beats/min is termed *sinus tachycardia.*

Regulation of the Heart Rate

The heart, like the other organs of the body, has a special nerve supply from the *autonomic nervous system,* which controls involuntary muscle action. The autonomic nerve supply to the heart (in particular, the SA and AV nodes) consists of two opposing groups of fibers: the *sympathetic nerves* and the *parasympathetic nerves.* Sympathetic stimulation produces an increased heart rate and also increases the strength of myocardial contraction. Parasympathetic stimulation (from the vagus nerve) produces a slowing of the heart rate as well as a slowing of conduction through the AV nodal area. In this way the autonomic nervous system exerts a counterbalancing control of the heart rate.

The sympathetic nervous system acts as a cardiac accelerator, whereas the parasympathetic (vagal) system produces a braking effect. For example, when you become excited or upset, increased sympathetic stimuli (and diminished parasympathetic tone) result in an increased heart rate and increased contractility, producing the familiar sensation of a pounding heart (palpitations).*

Sinus Tachycardia

Sinus tachycardia is simply sinus rhythm with a heart rate exceeding 100 beats/min. In adults the heart rate with sinus tachycardia is generally between 100 and 180 beats/min.

Fig. 11.2 shows an example of sinus tachycardia. Each QRS complex is preceded by a P wave. Notice that the P waves are positive in lead II. With sinus tachycardia at very fast rates the P wave may merge with the preceding T wave and become difficult to distinguish.

---

*Some authors define sinus bradycardia as a heart rate of less than 50 beats/min.

*Palpitations may be associated with a normal heartbeat, isolated premature beats (atrial or ventricular), or an actual run of ectopic (nonsinus) heartbeats (e.g., from atrial fibrillation, paroxysmal supraventricular tachycardia, or ventricular tachycardia).

In general, sinus tachycardia occurs with any condition that produces an *increase* in sympathetic tone or a *decrease* in vagal tone. The following conditions are commonly associated with sinus tachycardia:

- Anxiety, excitement, exertion, and pain
- Drugs that increase sympathetic tone (e.g., epinephrine, dopamine, tricyclic antidepressants, isoproterenol, and cocaine)
- Drugs that block vagal tone (e.g., atropine and other anticholinergic agents)

Normal Sinus Rhythm

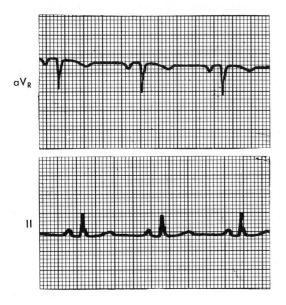

Fig. 11.1 Each QRS complex is preceded by a P wave that is negative in lead aV_R and positive in lead II.

- Fever, many infections, and septic shock
- Congestive heart failure (CHF) (Sinus tachycardia caused by increased sympathetic tone is generally seen with pulmonary edema.)
- Pulmonary embolism (As noted in Chapter 10, sinus tachycardia is the most common arrhythmia seen with acute pulmonary embolism.)
- Acute myocardial infarction (MI), which may produce virtually any arrhythmia (Sinus tachycardia persisting after an acute MI is generally a bad prognostic sign and implies extensive heart damage.)
- Hyperthyroidism (Sinus tachycardia occurring at rest may be an important diagnostic clue.)
- Intravascular volume loss because of bleeding, vomiting, diarrhea, pancreatitis, dehydration, and related conditions
- Alcohol intoxication or withdrawal

Treatment of sinus tachycardia associated with a pathologic condition must be directed at the underlying cause (e.g., infection, hyperthyroidism, CHF, or alcohol withdrawal).*

Sinus Bradycardia

With sinus bradycardia, sinus rhythm is present and the heart rate is less than 60 beats/min

---

*A small subset of patients who complain of palpitations (typically young adults) are found to have *inappropriate sinus tachycardia.* The causes of this syndrome are not certain. In some cases autonomic factors may play a role; in others a reentrant tachycardia originating in the SA node is discovered.

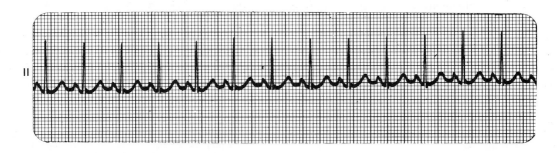

Fig. 11.2 Sinus tachycardia.

(Fig. 11.3). This arrhythmia commonly occurs in the following conditions:

- Normal variant (Many people have a resting pulse rate of less than 60 beats/min, and trained athletes may have a resting or sleeping pulse rate as low as 35 beats/min.)
- Drugs that increase vagal tone (e.g., digitalis or edrophonium) or that decrease sympathetic tone (e.g., beta blockers) (In addition, calcium channel blockers such as diltiazem and verapamil may cause marked sinus bradycardia.)
- Hypothyroidism
- Hyperkalemia
- Sick sinus syndrome (Some patients, particularly elderly ones, have marked sinus bradycardia without obvious cause, probably from degenerative disease of the SA node or surrounding tissue. Sick sinus syndrome is discussed further at the end of this chapter and in Chapter 18; see also Fig. 11.5.)
- Sleep apnea syndrome
- Carotid sinus hypersensitivity syndrome
- Vasovagal reactions

Moderate sinus bradycardia usually produces no symptoms. If the heart rate is very slow (i.e., 40 to 50 beats/min), light-headedness and even syncope may occur. Treatment requires decreasing medication doses or even discontinuing drug therapy (e.g., beta blockers or calcium channel blockers). If inappropriate sinus bradycardia causes symptoms (as in sick sinus syndrome), an electronic pacemaker may be needed (see Chapter 20).

Sinus Arrhythmia

Even in healthy people the SA node does not pace the heart at a perfectly regular rate, and a slight beat-to-beat variation is normally present (Fig. 11.4). When this variability is more accentuated, the term *sinus arrhythmia* is used.

The most common cause of sinus arrhythmia is respiration. *Respiratory sinus arrhythmia* is a

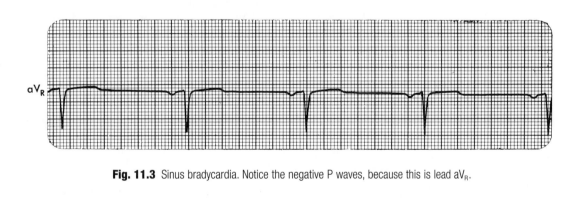

Fig. 11.3 Sinus bradycardia. Notice the negative P waves, because this is lead aV_R.

Fig. 11.4 Respiratory sinus arrhythmia. Normally the heart rate increases slightly with inspiration and decreases slightly with expiration.

normal finding and may be quite marked (up to 10 to 20 beats/min), particularly in children and young adults. The heart rate normally increases slightly with inspiration and decreases slightly with expiration because of changes in vagal tone that occur during the different phases of respiration (see Fig. 11.4).

Sinus Pauses, Sinus Arrest, and Escape Beats

Normal sinus rhythm, sinus tachycardia, sinus bradycardia, and sinus arrhythmia have been considered. Now suppose that the sinus node fails to stimulate the atria for one or more beats. Such dysfunction may occur intermittently, with simply a missed beat (no P wave or QRS complex) at occasional intervals, or it may be more extreme.* An example of the latter is *sinus pause* or *sinus arrest,* in which the SA node fails to stimulate the atria for a prolonged period (Fig. 11.5). This leads to cardiac arrest with asystole unless the sinus node regains function or some other pacemaker (escape pacemaker) takes over. Fortunately, other parts of the cardiac conduction system are capable of producing electrical stimuli and functioning as an escape pacemaker in these circumstances. *Escape beats* may come from the atria, the AV node, or the ventricles. Fig. 11.6 shows a junctional escape beat. (The characteristics of escape beats are described in Chapter 12.)

SA block or arrest can be caused by numerous factors, including the following:
- Hypoxia
- Myocardial ischemia or infarction
- Hyperkalemia
- Digitalis toxicity
- Toxic reactions to drugs such as beta blockers and calcium channel blockers (e.g., diltiazem and verapamil)

Particularly in elderly persons, the SA node may undergo degenerative changes, with periods of SA dysfunction and bradycardia leading at times

---

*The two distinct mechanisms for sinus node dysfunction are sinus pacemaker failure and SA block. The former is due to actual failure of the SA node to electrically fire (depolarize) for one or more beats. The latter results when the SA node fires but the impulse is apparently blocked from exiting the node and stimulating the atria. From a clinical viewpoint, distinguishing between SA pacemaker dysfunction and SA (exit) block is usually not essential.

SINUS PAUSE

Fig. 11.5 Sinus pause in a patient with sick sinus syndrome. The monitor lead shows sinus bradycardia with a long pause (about 2.4 seconds).

Fig. 11.6 This monitor strip shows a sinus pause interrupted by a junctional escape *(JE)* beat. The wide QRS complex is due to an underlying bundle branch block.

to light-headedness and syncope. The term *sick sinus syndrome* refers to this type of SA node dysfunction (see Figs. 11.5 and 18.13).

In summary, the term *arrhythmia* refers to any heart rhythm other than strictly normal sinus rhythm. Sinus bradycardia, sinus tachycardia, sinus arrhythmia, and SA block are all arrhythmias. However, sinus bradycardia at rest, sinus tachycardia with exercise, and respiratory sinus arrhythmia are all normal findings. In other settings, sinus bradycardia or sinus tachycardia, may be an important diagnostic clue (e.g., sinus tachycardia for pulmonary embolism and sinus bradycadia for hypothyroidism).

The next few chapters describe important arrhythmias in which the cardiac pacemaker is located *outside* the SA node—in the atria, AV junction, or ventricles.

Review

With *normal sinus rhythm* each heartbeat originates in the sinus (or sinoatrial [SA]) node. The P wave is always negative in lead aV_R and positive in lead II. The heart rate is between 60 and 100 beats/min.

The heart rate is greater than 100 beats/min with *sinus tachycardia* and is less than 60 beats/min with *sinus bradycardia.* Sinus bradycardia and sinus tachycardia have multiple causes, and both rhythms may occur normally.

Beat-to-beat variation of the sinus rate occurs with *sinus arrhythmia.* The rate variation is typically phasic with respiration *(respiratory sinus arrhythmia).* SA node dysfunction (because of either pacemaker cell failure or exit block) may lead to sinus pauses or, in extreme cases, SA *arrest.* Prolonged sinus arrest causes fatal asystole unless normal sinus rhythm resumes or *escape beats* from other foci in the atria, atrioventricular junction, or ventricles take over. SA dysfunction may be seen, particularly in elderly people, as a consequence of *sick sinus syndrome.* Digitalis toxicity or toxic reactions to other drugs (e.g., beta blockers, calcium channel blockers, amiodarone) must always be excluded in patients with marked sinus bradycardia, SA pauses, or sinus arrest.

Questions

1. Is normal sinus rhythm present in the ECG leads shown below?

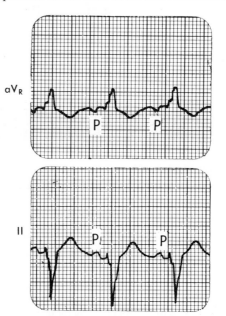

2. Is normal sinus rhythm present in this ECG lead?

Supraventricular Arrhythmias, Section I

Premature atrial and AV junctional beats, paroxysmal supraventricular tachycardias, and AV junctional rhythms

*T*he sinus node, or sinoatrial (SA) node, is the intrinsic pacemaker of the heart and normally initiates each heartbeat. However, pacemaker stimuli can arise from other parts of the heart, such as the atria, atrioventricular (AV) junction, or ventricles. The terms *ectopy, ectopic pacemaker,* and *ectopic beat* are used to describe these nonsinus heartbeats.

Ectopic beats are often premature; that is, they come before the next sinus beat is due. Thus *atrial premature beats (APBs), AV junctional premature beats (JPBs),* and *ventricular premature beats (VPBs)* may be found. Ectopic beats can also come after a pause in the normal rhythm, as in the case of AV junctional or ventricular *escape* beats. Ectopic beats originating in the AV junction (node) or atria are referred to as *supraventricular* (i.e., coming from *above* the ventricles).

In this chapter and the next, ectopic atrial and AV junctional (supraventricular) rhythms are described. Chapter 14 discusses ventricular ectopy.

Atrial and AV Junctional (Nodal) Premature Beats

APBs* result from ectopic stimuli; that is, these beats arise from somewhere in either the left or right atrium but not in the SA node. The atria therefore are depolarized from an ectopic site. After an atrial or junctional depolarization, the stimulus may spread normally through the His-Purkinje system into the ventricles. For this reason, ventricular depolarization (QRS complex) is generally not affected by APBs or JPBs.

APBs have the following major features (Figs. 12.1 to 12.3):
1. The atrial depolarization is premature, occurring before the next normal P wave is due.

---

*The terms *atrial premature contractions, atrial premature beats, atrial premature depolarizations,* and *atrial extrasystoles* are used synonymously. Most cardiologists prefer the designations *premature beat, depolarization,* and *complex* because not every premature stimulus is associated with an actual mechanical contraction of the atria or ventricles.

Fig. 12.1 A, Notice the atrial premature beat *(APB)* after the fourth sinus beat *(arrow).* **B,** Notice also the blocked atrial premature beat, again after the fourth sinus beat *(arrow).* The premature P wave falls on the T wave of the preceding beat and is not followed by a QRS complex because the atrioventricular node is still in a refractory state.

Fig. 12.2 Atrial bigeminy in which each sinus beat is followed by an atrial premature beat (or premature atrial complex).

2. The QRS complex of the APB is often preceded by a visible P wave that usually has a slightly different shape and/or different PR interval from the P wave seen with normal sinus beats. The PR interval of the APB may be either longer or shorter than the PR interval of the normal beats. In some cases the P wave may be "buried" in the T wave of the preceding beat.
3. After the APB a slight pause generally occurs before the normal sinus beat resumes.*
4. The QRS complex of the APB is usually identical or very similar to the QRS complex of the preceding beats. Remember that with APBs the atrial

pacemaker is in an ectopic location but the ventricles are usually depolarized in a normal way. This contrasts with VPBs, in which the QRS complex is usually very wide because of abnormal depolarization of the ventricles (see Chapter 14).

5. Occasionally, APBs result in aberrant ventricular conduction, so that the QRS complex is wider than normal. Fig. 12.3 shows an example of such beats causing delayed depolarization of the right ventricle. Thus these APBs are associated with right bundle branch block *aberrancy.* APBs with left bundle branch block aberrancy may also occur.
6. Sometimes when an APB is very premature, the stimulus reaches the AV junction just after it has been stimulated by the preceding normal

*This pause is due to "resetting" of the SA node pacemaker by the premature atrial stimulus.

Fig. 12.3 This rhythm strip shows sinus rhythm with three atrial premature beats. The first two (marked ●) are conducted with right bundle branch block aberrancy (rSR′ in lead V₁). The third atrial premature beat (○) is conducted with normal ventricular activation. Notice how the first two premature P waves come so early in the cardiac cycle that they fall on the T waves of the preceding sinus beats, making these T waves slightly taller.

beat. Because the AV junction, like all other conductive tissues, requires time to recover its capacity to conduct impulses, this premature atrial stimulus may reach the junction when it is still *refractory*. In this situation the APB may not be conducted to the ventricles and no QRS complex appears. The result is a *blocked* APB. The ECG shows a premature P wave *not* followed by a QRS complex (see Fig. 12.1, *B*). After the blocked P wave, a brief pause occurs before the next normal beat resumes. The blocked APB therefore produces a slight irregularity of the heartbeat. (If you do not search carefully for these blocked APBs, you may overlook them.)

The APBs may occur frequently (e.g., five or more times per minute) or sporadically. Two APBs occurring consecutively are referred to as an *atrial couplet*. Sometimes, as shown in Fig. 12.2, each sinus beat is followed by an APB. This pattern is referred to as *atrial bigeminy*.

CLINICAL SIGNIFICANCE

APBs are very common. They may occur with a normal heart or virtually any type of organic heart disease. Thus the presence of APBs does not imply that an individual has cardiac disease. In normal people these premature beats may

be seen with emotional stress, hyperthyroidism, excessive intake of caffeine, or the administration of sympathomimetic agents (epinephrine, isoproterenol, theophylline). APBs may produce palpitations; in this situation, patients may complain of feeling a skipped beat or an irregular pulse. APBs may also be seen with various types of structural heart disease. Frequent APBs are sometimes the forerunner of atrial fibrillation (see Chapter 13) or other atrial tachyarrhythmias.

Paroxysmal Supraventricular Tachycardias

Premature supraventricular beats may occur singly or repetitively. A sudden run of three or more beats constitutes a paroxysmal supraventricular tachycardia (PSVT). Episodes of PSVT may be brief and nonsustained (i.e., lasting from three beats up to 30 seconds). Sustained episodes (greater than 30 seconds) may last minutes, hours, or longer. The topic of PSVTs is actually quite complex. Therefore the following brief discussion is intended to provide only an introduction and overview.*

---

*See the Bibliography for texts that describe this important area of cardiology in more detail.

The three major types of PSVT are *atrial tachycardia (AT)* and related rhythms, *atrioventricular nodal reentrant tachycardia (AVNRT),* and *AV reentrant tachycardia (AVRT)* involving a bypass tract of the type seen in the Wolff-Parkinson-White (WPW) syndrome (see Chapter 10). These arrhythmias are depicted schematically in Fig. 12.4.

ATRIAL TACHYCARDIA (AT)

AT is defined simply as three or more consecutive APBs (Fig. 12.5). Most episodes appear to involve an ectopic (nonsinus) pacemaker located in either the left or right atrium that fires off "automatically" in a rapid way. A sustained episode lasting 30 seconds or longer, particularly at a rapid

Fig. 12.4 Major types of paroxysmal supraventricular tachycardia. **A,** The reference is normal sinus rhythm. **B,** With atrial tachycardia (AT), a focus *(X)* outside the sinoatrial *(SA)* node fires off automatically at a rapid rate. **C,** With atrioventricular *(AV)* nodal reentrant tachycardia (AVNRT) the cardiac stimulus originates as a wave of excitation that spins around the AV nodal (junctional) area. As a result, retrograde P waves may be buried in the QRS or appear immediately before or just after the QRS complex *(arrows)* because of nearly simultaneous activation of the atria and ventricles. **D,** A similar type of reentrant (circus-movement) mechanism may occur with a bypass tract *(BT)* of the type found in Wolff-Parkinson-White syndrome (see Fig. 10.20). This mechanism is referred to as *atrioventricular reentrant tachycardia.* Note the negative P wave *(arrow)* in lead II, somewhat after the QRS complex. (With AVRT the P wave in lead II may be negative, flat, or positive.)

rate, may cause light-headedness or even syncope (fainting) and in susceptible individuals can induce angina or congestive heart failure (CHF). The atrial rate with AT may be as high as 200 beats/min (range: 100 to 250 beats/min). AT has been observed in patients without apparent structural cardiac abnormality as well as in those with virtually any type of heart disease.* Short episodes may require no special therapy, but longer runs causing symptoms are usually treated initially with antiarrhythmic drugs.

AV NODAL REENTRANT TACHYCARDIA (AVNRT)

AVNRT, which was once mistakenly considered a variant of *paroxysmal atrial tachycardia*, is actually a distinct arrhythmia caused by a rapidly circulat-

---

*See Chapter 16 for a brief discussion of AT *with block* resulting from digitalis toxicity, and see Chapter 18 for a discussion of *multifocal atrial tachycardia (MAT)*.

ing impulse in the AV node area. The term *reentry* (introduced in Chapter 10) describes situations in which a cardiac impulse literally spins around and around and appears to "chase its own tail." Therefore, reentrant arrhythmias are sometimes referred to as *circus-movement* tachycardias. Reentry can occur in virtually any part of the heart. In the ventricles, for example, reentry leads to VPBs and sometimes ventricular tachycardia.

AVNRT produces a very rapid and regular supraventricular rhythm with rates typically between 140 and 250 beats/min (Fig. 12.6). This arrhythmia may occur with otherwise normal hearts or with underlying heart disease. Runs of AVNRT are generally initiated by an APB.

With AVNRT the reentrant rhythm originates in the AV nodal area and spreads simultaneously or nearly simultaneously up the atria and down the ventricles (see Fig. 12.4). As a consequence the P waves are usually hidden in the QRS complex because the atria and ventricles are activated

Fig. 12.5 Atrial tachycardia (a type of paroxysmal supraventricular tachycardia) terminating spontaneously with the abrupt resumption of sinus rhythm. The P waves of the tachycardia (rate: about 150 beats/min) are superimposed on the preceding T waves.

Paroxysmal Supraventricular Tachycardia

Fig. 12.6 Notice the marked regularity of rhythm in this paroxysmal supraventricular tachycardia *(PSVT)*, which has a rate of about 170 beats/min. This tachycardia is probably due to a rapidly circulating impulse in the atrioventricular (AV) node (junction) and thus is referred to as an *AV nodal reentrant tachycardia*. No P waves are visible (see also Fig. 12.4, *C*).

simultaneously. In other cases the P waves may appear just before or just after the QRS complex and therefore may be difficult to see. Because of this retrograde (bottom-to-top) activation of the atria, the P waves are negative in lead II. Episodes of AVNRT may cease spontaneously or may require treatment. The initial therapy usually involves attempts to increase vagal tone, since the vagus nerve slows conduction in the AV node. This "braking effect" may interrupt the reentrant mechanism (Fig. 12.7). Vagal tone can be increased with the Valsalva maneuver (i.e., the patient is instructed to strain against a closed glottis by bearing down, as for a bowel movement) or with carotid sinus massage.

A variety of drugs are used to interrupt the reentrant mechanism in AVNRT. Clinically, adenosine and verapamil are the drugs most often enlisted in the acute setting. Digoxin and beta blockers also are useful in selected cases.*

Younger patients and individuals without significant underlying cardiovascular disease may tolerate heart rates up to 250 beats/min with complaints of only palpitations or light-headedness. However, in patients with limited cardiac reserve a heart rate above 160 beats/min (or even less) can have disastrous consequences. In these patients,

myocardial ischemia or even infarction may occur. They may also develop CHF or hypotension. *Electrical cardioversion* may be required in emergency circumstances (i.e., when any PSVT is associated with angina, CHF, or severe hypotension and when initial therapy with vagal maneuvers and rapid-acting drugs fails).

Electrical cardioversion is the use of a direct-current (DC) shock to treat certain tachyarrhythmias.* The shock is administered with special paddles placed on the chest wall. An *unsynchronized* DC shock is used to treat some arrhythmias (e.g., ventricular flutter or ventricular fibrillation). However, a *synchronized* DC shock must be used to treat PSVT and other supraventricular arrhythmias (e.g., atrial fibrillation and atrial flutter). The shock is synchronized with the QRS complex so that it does not occur during the *vulnerable period* of ventricular repolarization (simultaneous with the apex of the T wave). Note that the DC shocks given to the heart during the vulnerable period may produce ventricular fibrillation. *Therefore, in treating PSVT, a synchronized DC shock must be given.*[†]

For patients with recurrent episodes of AVNRT, *radiofrequency (RF) catheter ablation* may be cura-

---

*Other drugs that may be used to interrupt the reentrant mechanism in AVNRT are discussed in various texts cited in the Bibliography.

---

*The electrical shock depolarizes the heart, interrupting abnormal rhythms and allowing the sinus node to "regain control" of the cardiac electrical cycle.

[†]For details on the use of electrical cardioversion to treat PSVT, see the appropriate texts cited in the Bibliography.

PSVT   Sinus rhythm

Carotid sinus massage

Fig. 12.7 Paroxysmal supraventricular tachycardia (PSVT) treated with carotid sinus massage. The first 14 beats in this rhythm strip show the tachyarrhythmia with a rate of about 140 beats/min and no visible P waves. Carotid sinus massage resulted in its abrupt termination, with the appearance of normal sinus rhythm. The PSVT here is probably an atrioventricular nodal reentrant tachycardia (AVNRT) (see Fig. 12.6).

tive. This special form of therapy, which is becoming increasingly widespread, involves delivering short pulses of RF current through an intracardiac catheter placed near the AV node during an electrophysiologic procedure. The current produces a very small burn that effectively blocks the part of the circuit that is supporting the reentrant-type wave.*

ATRIOVENTRICULAR REENTRANT (BYPASS TRACT) TACHYCARDIA (AVRT)

A third common cause of PSVT has already been introduced in the discussion of preexcitation syndromes (see Chapter 10). As previously mentioned, the WPW syndrome is related to the presence of a so-called *bypass tract* that connects the atria and ventricles, circumventing the AV node. Patients with this type of atrioventricular bypass tract may develop a tachycardia caused by a reentrant mechanism in which the impulse travels down the normal conduction system (AV node and His bundle) into the ventricles, recycles rapidly up into the atria via the bypass tract, and then goes down the AV node again. Repetition of this large reentrant circuit leads to a type of PSVT.

Of interest is the fact that in some patients the bypass tract is "concealed"; that is, it never becomes evident during sinus rhythm but functions only when a tachycardia starts.† The ECG with a concealed-bypass-tract type of PSVT is very similar to the ECG findings described for AVNRT. One subtle difference is that the ECGs of many patients with tachycardia associated with

a concealed bypass tract usually show P waves occurring shortly after the QRS complexes (see Fig. 12.5).

The therapy of PSVT resulting from a concealed bypass tract is quite similar to that of AVNRT. Drugs such as adenosine are used for acute episodes, and electrophysiologic testing is performed to evaluate the patient for possible RF catheter ablation of the bypass tract. Indeed, the most successful applications of RF ablation technology to date have been in the therapy of tachycardias associated with bypass tracts.

In summary, a PSVT should be suspected when a rhythm strip shows a rapid and typically very regular rate at about 200 beats/min (range: 100 to 250 beats/min). The mechanism may be due to reentry in the AV node (AVNRT), atrioventricular reentrant tachycardia (AVRT) with a concealed bypass tract, or ectopic AT. The differential diagnosis of PSVT and other supraventricular tachycardias is discussed further in Chapter 18.

AV Junctional Rhythms

With APVs the ectopic pacemaker is located somewhere in the atria outside the SA node. Under certain circumstances the AV junction may also function as an ectopic pacemaker, producing an AV junctional rhythm. In some discussions the term *AV nodal* or *nodal* is used to refer to an AV junctional rhythm. However, the terms *AV junctional, junctional, AV nodal,* and *nodal* are essentially synonymous.

Chapter 4 described the basic mechanism of AV junctional rhythms and the pattern seen with AV junctional escape beats. When the AV junction is the cardiac pacemaker, the atria are stimulated in a *retrograde* fashion, from bottom to top. An arrow representing the spread of atrial depolarization with junctional rhythm points upward, just opposite the direction of atrial depolarization when normal sinus rhythm is present (see Fig. 4.8). This retrograde stimulation of the atria produces a positive P wave in lead aV_R and a negative P wave in lead II (see Fig. 4.5). With AV junctional rhythm the ventricles are depolarized

---

*Consult texts cited in the Bibliography for more details on catheter ablation therapy for AVNRT and other arrhythmias.

†To be evident during sinus rhythm, the bypass tract must conduct impulses rapidly from the atria to the ventricles, bypassing the AV node. This produces a short PR interval, a wide QRS complex, and a delta wave—the classic triad of WPW preexcitation (see Fig. 10.20). In some patients with a bypass tract the pathway does not conduct antegrade very effectively, but it can still conduct retrograde under certain conditions, thereby allowing an impulse to reenter the atria from the ventricles. Bypass tracts that conduct only in a retrograde direction, causing PSVT, are said to be "concealed."

normally (unless a bundle branch block is present), resulting in a narrow QRS complex.

In some cases of AV junctional rhythm, the atria are stimulated just before the ventricles. In other cases the stimulus reaches the ventricles first. Finally, in many cases the atria and the ventricles are stimulated simultaneously. If the atria are stimulated first, the P wave precedes the QRS complex. (A retrograde P wave preceding the QRS complex also occurs with some ectopic atrial beats from the lower part of either atrium. However, the distinction between such "low" ectopic atrial and AV junctional beats is usually not of clinical importance.) If the ventricles are first to be stimulated, the QRS complex precedes the P wave. If atrial and ventricular depolarizations are simultaneous, the P wave is buried in the QRS and therefore is not seen.

In summary, AV junctional beats can be recognized on the ECG by one of the following patterns (Fig. 12.8):
- Retrograde P waves (positive in lead aV$_R$, negative in lead II) immediately preceding the QRS complexes
- Retrograde P waves immediately following the QRS complexes
- Absent P waves (buried in the QRS), so that the baseline between QRS complexes is flat

AV JUNCTIONAL ESCAPE RHYTHMS

AV junctional escape beats were mentioned in the discussion of sinus arrest (see Chapter 11). An AV junctional escape beat (Fig. 12.9) is simply a beat that comes after a pause when the normal sinus pacemaker fails to function. The AV junctional es-

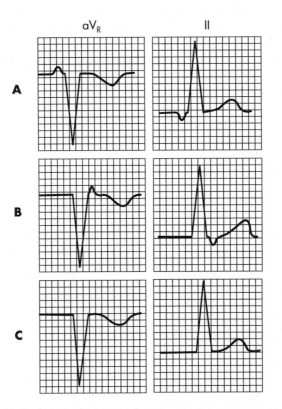

Fig. 12.8 Atrioventricular junctional (nodal) beats produce P waves that point upward in lead aV$_R$ and downward in lead II; this is just the opposite of what is seen with sinus rhythm. The P wave may just precede the QRS complex **(A),** follow it **(B),** or occur simultaneously with it **(C).** In the last instance no P wave is visible.

cape beat therefore is a "safety beat." After this escape beat, the normal sinus pacemaker may resume function. If it does not, a slow AV junctional escape rhythm may continue. An AV junctional escape rhythm is a consecutive run of AV junctional beats. The heart rate is usually slow (30 to 50 beats/min).

Fig. 12.10 shows an example of an AV junctional escape rhythm. Not surprisingly, the basic rate of the AV junction is slower than that of the SA node. If the AV junction had a faster inherent rate, it would compete with the SA node for control of the heartbeat.

AV junctional escape rhythms can be seen in a number of clinical settings, including digitalis toxicity (see Chapter 16), toxic reactions to beta blockers or calcium channel blockers (diltiazem and verapamil), acute myocardial infarction, hypoxemia, and hyperkalemia. The cause determines the treatment (e.g., stopping the digitalis or oxygenating the patient). If the heart rate becomes excessively slow with an AV junctional rhythm, drugs such as atropine (a vagal blocker) or isoproterenol (a sympathomimetic stimulant) may be used acutely to increase the heart rate.

As is true of AV junctional escape rhythms, *AV junctional tachycardias* can arise in a number of settings. Probably the most common type is AVNRT (see Fig. 12.4), an arrhythmia that results from a rapidly recirculating impulse in the nodal part of the AV junction. AV junctional tachycardias can also occur because of abnormally enhanced automaticity. This finding may, for example, occur with digitalis toxicity (see Chapter 16).*

---

*Additional information can be obtained from texts cited in the Bibliography.

Fig. 12.9 The junctional escape *(JE)* beat comes after a pause and is followed by a junctional premature complex *(JPC)*. Notice the retrograde (inverted) P wave preceding the JPB in this lead II rhythm strip.

Junctional Escape Rhythm

Fig. 12.10 This rhythm strip shows a slow junctional escape rhythm at about 40 beats/min. No P waves are visible, and the baseline between QRS complexes is flat.

Review

Stimuli that pace the heart can arise not only in the sinoatrial (SA) node but also in other cardiac tissues, such as the atria, atrioventricular (AV) junction, or ventricles. The terms *ectopy, ectopic pacemaker, ectopic contraction,* and *ectopic beat* are used to describe these stimuli. Ectopic beats can be divided into two major categories:

1. *Premature beats* are extra beats that come before the next normal beat is expected. Examples include *atrial premature beats (APBs), junctional premature beats,* and *ventricular premature beats.* These beats originate in the atria, AV junction, and ventricles, respectively.
2. *Escape beats* are usually AV junctional or ventricular beats that are *not* premature but come after a pause in the normal rhythm.

On ECGs, APBs show the following:

1. Usually, the P wave has a different shape, and the PR interval is slightly longer or shorter than in the preceding complexes. Sometimes the P wave is hidden in the T wave of the preceding normal beat.
2. Occasionally the atrial stimulus cannot penetrate the AV junction. In such cases of blocked APBs, the premature P wave is *not* followed by a QRS complex.

Paroxysmal ventricular tachycardia (PSVT) is a sudden run of three or more supraventricular beats. PSVT has three common types (see Fig. 12.4):

1. Atrial tachycardia (AT)
2. AV nodal reentrant tachycardia (AVNRT)
3. AV reentrant tachycardia (AVRT) associated with a bypass tract

AV junctional rhythms have the following features:

1. The P wave, when seen, is negative in lead II and positive in lead aV_R, which is just the reverse of the pattern seen with normal sinus rhythm. These are called *retrograde* P waves.
2. The retrograde P wave may immediately precede or follow the QRS complex.
3. In many cases the retrograde P wave is buried within the QRS complex. When this occurs, the baseline between QRS complexes remains completely flat.

AV junctional rhythms are categorized as *junctional escape rhythms* and *junctional tachycardias.* An AV junctional escape rhythm is a run of AV junctional beats with a slow rate, generally between 30 and 50 beats/min. AV junctional tachycardia, by contrast, is a more rapid run of three or more consecutive beats originating in the AV junction. A common type is AVNRT. Other types are due to increased automaticity of AV junctional pacemaker cells.

Questions

1. Based on the rhythm strip shown below, why might this patient complain of occasional palpitations?

V₁

2. What is the beat marked *X*?

3. Examine the rhythm strip shown below.
   a. What is the approximate heart rate?
   b. What class of arrhythmia is present?
      (1) Sinus tachycardia
      (2) Paroxysmal supraventricular tachycardia
      (3) Atrial flutter
      (4) Atrial fibrillation
      (5) Multifocal atrial tachycardia

Supraventricular Arrhythmias, Section II

Atrial flutter and atrial fibrillation

*A*trial flutter and *atrial fibrillation (AF)* (Fig. 13.1) are two distinct but related tachyarrhythmias. Like paroxysmal supraventricular tachycardia (PSVT), they are *ectopic*. In other words, with all three types of arrhythmias the atria are being stimulated *not* from the sinus, or sinoatrial (SA), node but from an ectopic site or sites. With PSVT the atria are stimulated at a rate generally between 140 and 250 beats/min. With atrial flutter the atrial rate is even faster, generally 250 to 350 beats/min. Finally, with AF the atrial depolarization rate is typically between 400 and 600 beats/min.*

With both atrial flutter and AF no discrete P waves are seen on the ECG. Instead, characteristic *flutter (F) waves* and *fibrillation (f) waves* represent continuous atrial electrical activity. Notice the pronounced "sawtooth" shape of the F waves and the rapid "tremulous" f waves in Fig. 13.1.

Atrial Flutter

With atrial flutter the stimulation rate is about 300 beats/min (Fig. 13.2). What happens to the ventricles during this rapid bombardment of the atria? The answer is that with atrial flutter (and atrial fibrillation) the ventricular (QRS) rate varies, depending on the ability of the atrioventricular (AV) junction to transmit stimuli from the atria to the ventricles. If the ventricles respond to each flutter wave, the ventricular rate is about 300 beats/min. Most commonly, the ventricular rate with atrial flutter is about 150, 100, or 75 beats/min. Atrial flutter with a ventricular response of 150 beats/min is called 2:1 flutter because the ratio of the atrial rate (300) to the ventricular rate (150) is 2 to 1. Atrial flutter with a ventricular rate of 100 beats/min is 3:1 flutter; with 75 beats/min it is usually 4:1 flutter. As mentioned, atrial flutter with a ventricular rate equal to the atrial rate (300 beats/min, or 1:1 flutter) is very rare. Characteristically, patients with atrial flutter increase or decrease their ventricular rate by stepwise fractions of the atrial rate (see Fig. 13.1). Thus a patient may change abruptly from atrial flutter with a ventricular response of 75 to 100 beats/min, to 150 beats/min or rarely even to 300 beats/min. In some patients the ventricular response with atrial flutter is more variable.*

---

*The QRS pattern of "group beating" is not uncommon with atrial flutter and represents a Wenckebach-type variant associated with bombardment of the AV node by frequent atrial depolarization waves (e.g., at 300 beats/min) (see Chapter 15).

It should also be noted that the atrial rate in atrial flutter may be considerably less than 250 beats/min (as low as 200 to 220 beats/min) in patients taking drugs that slow atrial conduction (e.g., quinidine, procainamide, amiodarone).

---

*The electrophysiologic mechanisms for the rapid reentrant waves that underlie atrial flutter and fibrillation are the subject of ongoing investigations (see the Bibliography).

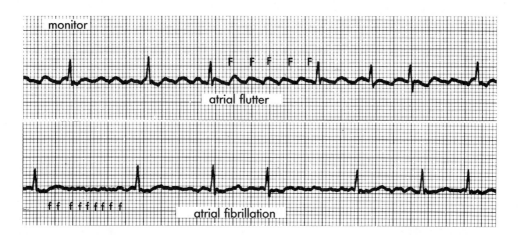

Fig. 13.1 Atrial flutter and fibrillation. Notice the "sawtooth" waves (*F* waves) with atrial flutter and the irregular fibrillatory waves (*f* waves) with atrial fibrillation.

Atrial Flutter

Fig. 13.2 A, Notice the variable appearance of flutter waves in different leads. In lead I the waves are barely apparent, whereas in leads II and III the classic "sawtooth" waves appear. The ventricular rate is about 160 beats/min, and the flutter rate is about 320 beats/min; thus 2:1 conduction is present. **B,** Carotid sinus massage produces marked slowing of the ventricular rate by increasing vagal tone.

CLINICAL SIGNIFICANCE

Atrial flutter is rarely seen in people with normal hearts. This is in contrast to AF, which may occur in normal individuals. Atrial flutter is not specific for any particular type of heart disease but occurs, for example, in patients with valvular heart disease, acute myocardial infarction (MI), chronic ischemic heart disease, cardiomyopathy, hypertensive heart disease, lung disease, and pulmonary emboli. It also occurs after cardiac surgery.

TREATMENT CONSIDERATIONS

The treatment of atrial flutter depends on the clinical condition. In some patients, atrial flutter may revert spontaneously to normal sinus rhythm. In patients who are hypoxic, oxygen therapy may help restore normal sinus rhythm.

Patients who have atrial flutter with a rapid ventricular response are usually treated initially with one drug or a combination of drugs (beta blockers, calcium channel blockers, digitalis) to slow impulse conduction through the AV node. Occasionally the arrhythmia converts to normal sinus rhythm spontaneously in the course of this initial therapy. In other cases a second drug (e.g., quinidine, procainamide, amiodarone, etc.) is added to help convert the flutter to normal sinus rhythm.

Despite initial therapy, atrial flutter persists in many patients. Fortunately, it is one of the arrhythmias most easily treated with direct current (DC) electrical cardioversion. As described in Chapter 12, a *synchronized* DC shock is given with the patient properly anesthetized.

In recent years radiofrequency (RF) catheter ablation has been used successfully to treat pa-tients with atrial flutter. Another way of attempting to convert atrial flutter is with very rapid pacing of the atria by means of a temporary pacing wire (known as *overdrive pacing*). This therapy may be particularly useful shortly after cardiac surgery when electrical pacing wires are still in place.

In summary, atrial flutter is a tachyarrhythmia in which the atria are stimulated (depolarized) at a rate of usually 250 to 350 beats/min, with a ventricular response that is often some fraction of the atrial rate ($\frac{1}{2}$, $\frac{1}{4}$, etc.). Atrial flutter may be treated with special drugs, synchronized DC shock, rapid atrial pacing, or RF ablation techniques.

Atrial Fibrillation

With AF, one of the most commonly seen arrhythmias, the atria are stimulated (depolarized) at a very rapid rate, up to 600 beats/min. This fibrillatory activity produces a characteristically irregular wavy pattern in place of the normal P waves. The irregular waves are called *fibrillatory* or *f waves* (Fig. 13.3). In some cases the f waves are relatively coarse (Fig. 13.4); in others a fine fibrillation is seen (Fig. 13.5). Therefore AF is characterized by rapid oscillatory depolarization of the atria that produces irregular undulations of the ECG baseline without discrete P waves.

Because of the rapid atrial depolarization rate, the AV junction in patients with AF is bombarded by innumerable stimuli from the atria. If every stimulus (each f wave) penetrated the AV junction, the ventricles would beat at a rate of up to 600 times per minute, with obvious conse-

Fig. 13.3 Rapid undulation of the baseline due to fibrillatory (f) waves. No true P waves are present, and the ventricular rate is irregular.

quences to the patient. Fortunately the AV junction is refractory to most of these impulses and allows only a fraction to reach the ventricles. In patients with a normal AV junction in whom AF suddenly develops, the ventricular rate is generally between 110 and 180 beats/min.* Fig. 13.5 shows an example of AF with a ventricular rate of about 140 beats/min. Characteristically the ventricular rate with AF is haphazardly irregular because the AV junction is being stimulated in an

---

*Always consider factors such as hypoxemia, severe anemia, fever, congestive heart failure, and hyperthyroidism, which can contribute to the rapid ventricular response and which, until corrected, may make rate control much more difficult.

apparently random fashion by the rapidly fibrillating atria.

In summary, AF has two ECG characteristics:
- An irregular wavy baseline produced by the rapid f waves
- A ventricular (QRS) rate that is usually quite irregular.

When the ventricular rate is very fast (Fig. 13.6), the f waves may be difficult to distinguish. In such cases the diagnosis of AF can usually be made by finding a very irregular ventricular rate in the absence of distinct P waves.

GENERAL CLINICAL ASPECTS

In some patients, AF occurs *paroxysmally* and may last only minutes, hours, or days. Some patients

Atrial Fibrillation with Rapid Response

Fig. 13.4 Coarse atrial fibrillatory waves with a rapid ventricular response. This patient has hyperthyroidism. (The commonly used term *rapid atrial fibrillation* is actually a misnomer, because "rapid" is intended to refer to the ventricular rate rather than the atrial rate. The same is true for the term *slow atrial fibrillation.*)

Atrial Fibrillation

Fig. 13.5 Fibrillatory waves may be hard to find. In this tachyarrhythmia no atrial waves are evident. The ventricular rate is about 140 beats/min and is irregular. No clear fibrillatory waves are visible; nevertheless, the rhythm is atrial fibrillation.

Atrial Fibrillation

Fig. 13.6 Relatively subtle fibrillation waves give the baseline between irregularly spaced R waves a wrinkly appearance.

may experience only one episode or occasional episodes, whereas others have multiple recurrences. In other patients, AF is *chronic* and may persist indefinitely. With these fibrillatory episodes, some patients are quite symptomatic (typically complaining of palpitations, weakness, or dyspnea), whereas others have no specific complaints. In the asymptomatic patient, AF may first be discovered during a routine examination or when the patient presents with heart failure or stroke.

AF can occur in normal persons and in patients with a variety of cardiac diseases (see Chapter 22). The term *lone atrial fibrillation* is sometimes used to describe recurrent or chronic AF in patients without other clinical evidence of heart disease. Paroxysmal AF may occur spontaneously, or it may be associated with excessive alcohol consumption in otherwise healthy individuals ("holiday heart syndrome"). In such cases, the arrhythmia often spontaneously reverts to normal sinus rhythm or is converted easily with pharmacologic therapy alone.

Changes in autonomic tone may provoke AF in susceptible individuals. Sometimes the arrhythmia is related to excessive sympathetic tone (e.g., occurring during exercise or with emotional excitement). At other times, AF may occur in the context of high vagal tone (e.g., with sinus bradycardia during sleep).

AF is also one of the most frequently observed arrhythmias in patients with organic (structural) heart disease. The prevalence of this arrhythmia rises with advancing age. Common pathologic substrates include coronary artery disease, hypertensive heart disease, and valvular heart disease. Patients with coronary artery disease may experience AF for the first time during an acute MI or as a consequence of chronic ischemic myocardial disease, presumably because of associated atrial dilation or fibrosis. Hypertensive heart disease is often associated with left atrial enlargement. AF is also commonly caused by valvular heart disease, particularly when the mitral valve is involved. For example, severe mitral stenosis or mitral regurgitation produces atrial enlargement, which is a predisposing factor for atrial arrhythmias.

Numerous other conditions can also lead to AF. For example, patients with thyrotoxicosis (hyperthyroidism) may develop AF (see Fig. 13.5). AF (or atrial flutter) is not uncommon after cardiac surgery. It may also occur with pericardial disease (especially chronic disease), lung disease, pulmonary emboli, cardiomyopathy, congenital heart disease (e.g., atrial septal defect), and other forms of heart disease. Often, patients have more than one predisposing factor for this arrhythmia.

CLINICAL CONSEQUENCES

What happens physiologically when AF develops? After the P wave the atria normally contract and pump blood into the ventricles. With AF, normal atrial depolarization is lost and the atria fibrillate (quiver) instead of contracting synchronously. In these circumstances the normal atrial "kick" is lost, and the result is decreased cardiac output (since ventricular filling is decreased) and sometimes thromboembolization.

Decreased Cardiac Output

Hemodynamically the most significant effect of AF is decreased cardiac output, which is especially marked in patients with underlying cardiac impairment and in elderly people, who appear to be more dependent on atrial contraction for filling of the ventricles. In addition, the amount of this decreased output depends on the ventricular rate with AF. The faster the rate, the more decreased the cardiac output becomes. Thus the patient with AF at a rate of 180 beats/min is more likely to be hypotensive or in congestive heart failure (CHF) than is the patient with a rate of 100 beats/min. In patients with coronary artery disease this rapid ventricular rate can cause myocardial ischemia and even infarction (see Chapter 8).

Atrial Thrombi and Embolization

The second significant effect of AF, resulting from the stagnation of blood, is a tendency in some patients for atrial thrombi to develop and dislodge into the arterial circulation, causing peripheral embolism. The thrombi can produce a cerebrovascular accident, occlusion of the blood supply to the legs, and other complications.

The risk of thrombus formation and embolization is highest in patients with chronic AF related to rheumatic mitral valve disease. However, thrombi and embolization also occur in patients with AF from other causes (so-called *nonrheumatic atrial fibrillation*). Indeed, *atrial fibrillation is a major substrate for embolic strokes, particularly in the elderly.*

TREATMENT

Rather than discussing the details of treating AF, this section focuses on the general clinical approach to patients with this arrhythmia. AF is converted to sinus rhythm in two principal ways. The first is with *pharmacologic* therapy. The second is with *electrical cardioversion* (as described for PSVT and atrial flutter).

In approaching patients with AF, you need to answer at least four major clinical questions:
1. Is the arrhythmia causing a life-threatening decrease in cardiac function, as indicated by myocardial ischemia, hypotension, or CHF? As a general rule, patients with very recent-onset AF that is producing myocardial ischemia, shock, or pulmonary edema should be considered candidates for electrical cardioversion if they do not respond promptly to drug therapy.
2. Is the AF acute or chronic?
3. Does the patient require short- or long-term anticoagulation?
4. What is the cause of the arrhythmia?

In most cases, acute paroxysmal AF does not require immediate electrical cardioversion. Drug therapy alone can be used initially to control the ventricular rate. Beta blockers, calcium channel blockers (verapamil, diltiazem), and digitalis all act by slowing conduction of stimuli through the AV node.*

The usual sequence in treating AF pharmacologically is to slow the ventricular response with a beta blocker, calcium channel blocker, or digitalis. If sinus rhythm is not restored after rate slowing, the addition of an antiarrhythmic drug is often considered.† Elective DC cardioversion is generally reserved for patients who fail to respond to an initial trial of drug therapy.

Attempts to convert AF to sinus rhythm with either pharmacologic therapy or DC cardioversion should not be made unless the patient has been sufficiently anticoagulated or atrial thrombus formation has been convincingly excluded (e.g., by transesophageal echocardiography). The reason for this caveat is that restoration of normal atrial contractility during sinus rhythm may cause dislodgment of an atrial thrombus formed

---

*Digitalis acts primarily by increasing vagal tone. Beta blockers decrease sympathetic tone. Calcium channel blockers directly interfere with conduction by impairing the cellular entry of calcium ions, which play a major role in electrical impulse transmission in the AV node.

†The decisions on whether to add an antiarrhythmic agent for pharmacologic conversion and the specific drug to use are complex and controversial. See the Bibliography for texts that provide in-depth discussions of these issues.

during the fibrillation. The longer the duration of the fibrillation, the more likely thrombus formation becomes. However, thrombus formation may also occur with fibrillation of relatively short duration. Patients with chronic or paroxysmal AF that cannot be converted to sinus rhythm are candidates for long-term anticoagulation with warfarin or aspirin, depending on the circumstances.*

Some patients with chronic AF that cannot be converted to sinus rhythm have an uncontrollably fast ventricular response despite intensive drug therapy. A relatively new approach to this problem is ablation of the AV node with RF current delivered by a special cardiac catheter (see Chapter 12). Because this therapy often results in complete heart block, a permanent pacemaker must also be implanted.

At the same time that you are starting to treat a patient with AF, you should be thinking of

---

*Current guidelines for specific anticoagulation regimens before and after attempted cardioversion in paroxysmal or chronic AF are provided in texts cited in the Bibliography.

possible causes for this arrhythmia. You should search for evidence of excessive alcohol use (holiday heart syndrome), hypertensive heart disease, cardiomyopathy, valvular disease, coronary artery disease, or pericardial disease. A blood test for thyroid function should be performed in any patient with unexplained AF because thyrotoxicosis is an important treatable cause of this arrhythmia.

Patients with underlying AV nodal disease may develop AF with a slow ventricular response in the absence of drug therapy. If the ventricular rate becomes exceedingly slow, a permanent pacemaker may be required.

ATRIAL FIBRILLATION AND OTHER ARRHYTHMIAS

AF (or atrial flutter) may occur with other arrhythmias and conduction disturbances, just as sinus rhythm can occur with ventricular premature beats (VPBs), AV heart block, and so on. An example of AF with VPBs is presented in Fig. 13.7. AF or atrial flutter can also occur with complete

Fig. 13.7 Atrial fibrillation with ventricular premature beats.

Fig. 13.8 Atrial fibrillation with complete atrioventricular block. The ventricular rate is very slow and regular because of the block. (Notice the right bundle branch block morphology of the escape rhythm QRS complexes.)

heart block (Fig. 13.8); in such cases the ventricular response is very slow and regular. Possible digitalis toxicity should always be considered in the patient who has AF and a very slow ventricular rate (see Chapter 16).

AF with the Wolff-Parkinson-White syndrome is discussed in Chapter 18.

Occasionally it can be difficult to decide whether AF or atrial flutter is present (see Chapter 19). The coarse atrial fibrillatory waves may resemble flutter waves (see Fig. 19.3). This arrhythmia, which is sometimes referred to as *flutter-fibrillation,* has the same clinical significance and treatment as atrial fibrillation.

Review

With *atrial flutter,* the ECG shows the following:

1. Characteristic "sawtooth" flutter waves instead of discrete P waves
2. A constant or variable ventricular rate (e.g., one QRS complex with every fourth flutter wave, 4:1 flutter; one QRS with every two flutter waves, 2:1 flutter, and the ventricular rate half the atrial rate; or the rare 1:1 flutter, in which the ventricles contract about 300 times a minute)

Atrial flutter rarely occurs in normal hearts but is most often seen in valvular heart disease, ischemic heart disease, lung disease, cardiomyopathy, or pulmonary emboli. It may also occur after cardiac surgery. Atrial flutter may be treated with a synchronized direct-current (DC) shock (cardioversion), drug therapy, rapid atrial pacing, or radiofrequency catheter ablation.

The ECG of a patient with *atrial fibrillation (AF)* shows the following:

1. Rapid irregular undulations of the baseline (fibrillatory waves) instead of P waves
2. A ventricular rate that is usually grossly irregular

In some patients AF occurs chronically; in others it is paroxysmal. Occasionally, AF is seen in healthy people. Common causes are coronary artery disease, hypertensive heart disease, and mitral valve disease. This arrhythmia may also occur with hyperthyroidism, cardiomyopathy, excessive alcohol use, cardiac surgery, pulmonary emboli, and chronic pericarditis. It may be seen with other arrhythmias (e.g., ventricular ectopy or complete heart block). With an extremely slow ventricular rate (50 beats/min or less), AF may signify digitalis toxicity. Sustained AF sometimes can be converted to normal sinus rhythm with DC cardioversion or pharmacologic therapy.

Questions

1. Answer the following questions about the monitor lead rhythm strip below:
   a. What is the atrial rate?
   b. What is the ventricular rate?
   c. What is this arrhythmia?

2. Answer the following questions about this rhythm strip:
   a. What is the *average* heart rate?
   b. What is the rhythm?

II

3. The atrial rate with atrial flutter is *(faster, slower)* than the atrial rate with atrial fibrillation.
4. The atrial rate with atrial flutter is *(faster, slower)* than that with atrial tachycardia.
5. The ventricular rate with atrial fibrillation is always greater than 100 beats/min *(true or false)*.

Ventricular Arrhythmias

The three preceding chapters have focused on *supra*ventricular arrhythmias, which are rhythm disturbances arising in the sinus node, atria, or atrioventricular (AV) junction with normal ventricular depolarization. This chapter considers another major ECG topic—ventricular arrhythmias. Ectopic (nonsinus) beats frequently arise in the ventricles themselves, producing *premature ventricular beats (or complexes), ventricular tachycardia (VT)*, and sometimes *ventricular fibrillation (VF)*.

Ventricular Premature Beats

Ventricular premature beats (VPBs)* are premature depolarizations arising in the ventricles, analogous to atrial premature beats (APBs) and junctional premature beats (JPBs), which are supraventricular. Recall that with APBs and JPBs the QRS complex is usually of normal width because the stimulus spreads normally through the bundle branches to the ventricles. With VPBs, however, the premature depolarizations arise in either the right or left ventricle. Therefore the ventricles are not stimulated simultaneously, and the stimulus spreads through the ventricles in an aberrant direction. Thus the QRS complexes are wide with VPBs, just as they are with the bundle branch block patterns. Examples of VPBs are shown in Figs. 14.1 to 14.8.

---

*In the ECG literature the terms *ventricular premature beat, ventricular premature depolarization, ventricular extrasystole,* and *premature ventricular complex* or *contraction (PVC)* are used interchangeably.

VPBs have two major characteristics*:
1. They are premature and occur before the next normal beat is expected.
2. They are aberrant in appearance. The QRS complex is abnormally wide (usually 0.12 second or more), and the T wave and QRS complex usually point in opposite directions.

VPBs usually precede a sinus P wave. Occasionally they appear just after a sinus P wave but before the normal QRS complex (see Fig. 14.7). Sometimes they are followed by a nonsinus P wave (negative in lead II) that has arisen because of retrograde stimulation of the atria by the VPB.

FEATURES
Clinicians tend to comment on a number of features of VPBs that may have clinical relevance.

Frequency
The frequency of VPBs refers to the number that are seen per minute or other unit of time. The VPB frequency may range from one or an occasional isolated premature depolarization to many.

VPBs may occur in various combinations. Two in a row (see Fig. 14.4) are referred to as a *pair* or *couplet*. Three or more in a row are, by definition, VT (see Fig. 14.5). Sometimes, as shown in

---

*The basic electrophysiologic mechanisms responsible for VPBs are a subject of active investigation. VPBs may arise by at least three mechanisms: *reentrant waves,* increased *spontaneous depolarizations* of ventricular cells (enhanced automaticity), and *triggered activity* or *afterdepolarizations* (i.e., premature firing of ventricular cells triggered by the previous depolarization).

Fig. 14.1 A ventricular premature beat *(VPB)* is recognized because it comes before the next normal beat is expected and it has a wide aberrant shape. Notice also the long PR interval in the normal sinus beats, indicating first-degree atrioventricular block.

Fig. 14.2 Notice the wide aberrant shape of a ventricular premature beat *(VPB)* compared to the QRS complexes of an atrial premature beat *(APB)*, which generally resembles the sinus QRS complexes.

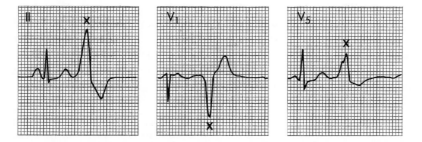

Fig. 14.3 Notice that the same ventricular premature beat (marked X) recorded simultaneously in three different leads has different shapes. By comparison, notice that the multiform ventricular premature beats shown in Fig. 14.9 have different shapes in the *same* lead.

Monitor lead

Fig. 14.4 Two ventricular premature beats *(V)* are referred to as a *pair* or a *couplet.* They also show the "R on T" phenomenon (see text and Fig. 14.10) (*P,* P wave; *T,* T wave).

Nonsustained Ventricular Tachycardia

Fig. 14.5 Notice the two short bursts of *nonsustained ventricular tachycardia (VT).* Compare this with the sustained VT shown in Fig. 14.12, *A.*

Fig. 14.6 A, Ventricular bigeminy, in which each normal sinus impulse is followed by a ventricular premature beat (marked X). **B,** Ventricular trigeminy, in which a ventricular premature beat occurs after every two sinus pulses.

Fully Compensatory Pause

Fig. 14.7 Some ventricular premature beats *(VPB)* cause a fully compensatory pause, with the interval between the two sinus beats that surround the VPB (R_3 and R_4 in this case) being exactly two times the normal interval between sinus beats (R_1 and R_2). Notice that the P waves *(P)* come on time, except that the third P wave is interrupted by the VPB and therefore is not conducted through the atrioventricular junction, which is still refractory. The next (fourth) P wave also comes on time. The fact that the sinus node is continuing to pace despite the VPB results in the fully compensatory pause.

Interpolated Ventricular Premature Beats

Fig. 14.8 Sometimes a ventricular premature beat *(X)* falls between two normal beats, in which case it is *interpolated.*

Fig. 14.6, *A,* isolated VPBs occur so frequently that each normal beat is followed by a VPB. This produces a distinctive repetitive grouping of one normal beat and one VPB, which is called *ventricular bigeminy.* The sequence of two normal beats with a VPB is *ventricular trigeminy.*

Coupling Interval

The term *coupling interval* is frequently applied to the interval between the VPB and the preceding normal beat. When multiple VPBs are present, *fixed coupling* often occurs, with the coupling interval approximately the same for each VPB (see

Fig. 14.6). At other times, VPBs may show a *variable coupling interval.*

Compensatory Pause

As you may have noticed, APBs and VPBs are usually followed by a pause before the next normal beat. The pause after a VPB is usually but not always longer than the pause after an APB. A fully compensatory pause indicates that the interval between the normal QRS complexes immediately before and immediately after the VPB is exactly twice the basic RR interval (see Fig. 14.7). A fully compensatory pause is more characteristic

Multiform Ventricular Premature Beats

II

VPB   VPB   VPB

Fig. 14.9 These multiform ventricular premature beats *(VPB)* have different shapes in the same lead. (Compare this tracing with the one in Fig. 14.3.)

Monitor lead

X

Fig. 14.10 A ventricular premature beat (*X*) falling near the peak of the T wave of the preceding beat may be a predisposing factor for ventricular tachycardia or ventricular fibrillation, particularly when this "R on T" phenomenon occurs in the setting of acute myocardial ischemia or infarction or with long QT(U) intervals.

of VPBs than APBs. Sometimes a VPB falls almost exactly between two normal beats; in such cases the VPB is said to be *interpolated* (see Fig. 14.8).

Uniform and Multiform VPBs

The terms *uniform* and *multiform* are used to describe the appearance of VPBs in any lead. Uniform VPBs have the same appearance in any lead and arise from the same anatomic site (focus) (see Fig. 14.6). (Of course, they have different shapes in different leads, just as normal beats do.) By contrast, multiform VPBs have different morphologies in the same lead (Fig. 14.9). Multiform VPBs often but not always arise from different foci. Uniform VPBs are uni*focal,* but multi*form* VPBs are not nec-

essarily multi*focal.* Uniform VPBs may occur in normal hearts and hearts with underlying organic heart disease. Multiform VPBs usually indicate that organic heart disease is present.

R on T Phenomenon

The *R on T* or *VPB on T phenomenon* refers to VPBs that are timed so that they fall near the peak* of the T wave of the preceding normal beat (see Figs. 14.10 and 14.16). Those falling on the T wave are noteworthy in that they may precipitate VT or

___
*Alternatively, the VPBs may fall at the nadir of a negative T wave.

VF, particularly in the course of an acute myocardial infarction (MI) or myocardial ischemia or with very long QT intervals (discussed later in this chapter). Recall from the discussion of synchronized direct-current (DC) cardioversion that the peak of the T wave is a time during which an external stimulus is especially likely to produce VF (see Chapter 12). However, VT and VF most commonly occur without a preceding "R on T" beat, and most "R on T" beats do not precipitate a sustained ventricular tachyarrhythmia.

CLINICAL SIGNIFICANCE

VPBs are among the most common arrhythmias. They may occur in normal hearts and with serious organic heart disease. Individuals with VPBs may be asymptomatic, or they may complain of palpitations (i.e., sensations of a "skipped" or "extra" beat). VPBs may be a stable and benign finding, or they may be a marker of severe organic heart disease associated with an increased risk of cardiac arrest and sudden death from VF. Clearly, clinicians need certain ground rules to help decide when VPBs are of concern. A few general principles are discussed here.

As mentioned, VPBs are not uncommon in normal adults of all ages although they occur more frequently with advancing age. Young adults, for example, may have VPBs because of anxiety or excessive caffeine intake. Certain drugs used in asthmatics (e.g., epinephrine, isoproterenol, and aminophylline) can provoke VPBs in normal hearts. Nevertheless, if a patient has frequent VPBs, you should search carefully for underlying cardiac disease (heart murmurs, abnormal echocardiographic findings, etc.) and also obtain a careful drug history. Occasional or even frequent isolated VPBs in an otherwise healthy person without organic heart disease are not usually a source of concern. VPBs are also common with mitral valve prolapse, and they may be seen with virtually any type of heart disease. For example, a patient with valvular, hypertensive, or ischemic heart disease with or without MI may have them. VPBs are the most common arrhythmia seen with acute MI.

As noted, VPBs can be caused by the effects on the heart of numerous drugs, including epineph-rine, isoproterenol, and aminophylline, which are cardiac stimulants. Ventricular ectopy is also an important sign of digitalis toxicity (see Chapter 16). VPBs may be seen in patients with electrolyte disturbances such as hypokalemia or hypomagnesemia and in patients with lung disease or hypoxemia from any cause.

DRUG THERAPY

As mentioned, VPBs are common in healthy people. Even in patients with underlying heart disease the suppression of frequent isolated VPBs or even short runs of VT with antiarrhythmic drugs has not been shown to improve survival. In fact, the drugs used to treat ventricular ectopy (e.g., quinidine, procainamide, disopyramide, mexiletine, propafenone, moricizine, and flecainide) all have grave and sometimes life-threatening side effects. Furthermore, antiarrhythmic drugs may actually make the situation worse by increasing the severity of the ectopy (*proarrhythmic effect*). Indeed, treating a patient with so-called *antiarrhythmic* drugs may sometimes provoke a potentially fatal ventricular tachyarrhythmia.*

For patients with frequent VPBs associated with very bothersome palpitations, beta-blocker therapy is sometimes used. Beta blockers may also be helpful in patients who have ventricular ectopy associated with coronary artery disease and in patients who have certain types of cardiomyopathy.

These complex and sometimes controversial therapeutic issues are discussed more completely in texts cited in the Bibliography. Again, *whenever you see a patient with frequent VPBs, you must search for potentially reversible causes, particularly hypokalemia, hypomagnesemia, and certain drugs.*

Ventricular Tachycardia

VT is, by definition, simply a run of three or more consecutive VPBs. Examples are shown in Figs. 14.5, 14.11, and 14.12. VT is usefully

---

*Consult the Bibliography for a discussion of the Cardiac Arrhythmia Suppression Trial (CAST study), which demonstrated the life-threatening proarrhythmic effects of certain drugs in patients with prior MI.

Paroxysmal Nonsustained Ventricular Tachycardia

Monitor - continuous strip

Fig. 14.11 The monitor lead shows short bursts of ventricular tachycardia.

Sustained, Monomorphic Ventricular Tachycardia Terminated by Direct-Current Shock

DC shock

A

B

Fig. 14.12 A, Long run of monomorphic ventricular tachycardia. **B,** Normal sinus rhythm restored after direct-current *(DC)* cardioversion.

Ventricular Fibrillation

Fig. 14.13 Ventricular fibrillation *(VF)* may produce both coarse and fine waves. Immediate defibrillation should be performed.

Cardiac Arrest

Fig. 14.14 Ventricular tachycardia *(VT)* and ventricular fibrillation *(VF)* recorded during the onset of cardiac arrest. The rapid sine-wave type of VT seen here is sometimes referred to as *ventricular flutter.*

classified by duration (nonsustained and sustained) and by morphology (monomorphic and polymorphic) (box).

Sustained VT (typically lasting more than 30 seconds) is usually a life-threatening arrhythmia for two major reasons:

1. Most patients are not able to maintain an adequate blood pressure at very rapid ventricular rates and eventually become hypotensive.
2. The condition may degenerate into VF (see Fig. 14.13), causing immediate cardiac arrest.

VT, whether sustained or not, can also be characterized as *monomorphic* (see Fig. 14.12, *A*) or *polymorphic* (see Fig. 14.16), depending on whether consecutive VPBs have the same or a variable appearance in a single lead. Very rapid VT with a sine-wave appearance is sometimes referred to as *ventricular flutter.* This arrhythmia often leads to VF (Fig. 14.14).

CAUSES AND THERAPY OF RECURRENT, SUSTAINED, MONOMORPHIC VENTRICULAR TACHYCARDIA

Sustained VT, which may lead to syncope or sudden death, rarely occurs in patients without underlying structural heart disease.* Most patients with this type of high-grade ventricular ectopy (i.e., long runs of ventricular tachycardia) have some basic structural cardiac abnormality, such as prior MI, cardiomyopathy or valvular disease associated with fibrosis (scarring), or ventricular enlargement. The most common cause of sustained monomorphic VT in American adults is coronary artery disease with prior MI.

---

*See texts cited in the Bibliography for discussions of the types of VT that may occur *without* structural heart disease.

Accelerated Idioventricular Rhythm

aV_F-Continuous strip

Fig. 14.15 Accelerated idioventricular rhythm (AIVR) in a patient with an acute inferior wall infarction. The first four beats show the typical pattern, followed by a return of sinus rhythm, then the reappearance of the AIVR. Notice that the fifth, sixth, twelfth, and thirteenth QRS complexes are "fusion beats" because of the nearly simultaneous occurrence of a sinus beat and a ventricular beat (*P, P* wave).

Despite pharmacologic therapy, some patients are at high risk for life-threatening recurrences of sustained VT or VF. For these patients a special device called an *implantable cardioverter defibrillator (ICD)* has been developed to deliver an electric shock directly to the heart during a life-threatening tachycardia.*

Accelerated Idioventricular Rhythm

Figs. 14.15 and 14.16 present a distinctive arrhythmia that has been called *accelerated idioventricular rhythm (AIVR)* or *slow ventricular tachycardia*. Recall that with typical VT the heart rate is faster than 100 beats/min. With AIVR the heart rate is usually between 50 and 100 beats/min, and the ECG shows wide QRS complexes without associated P waves.

AIVR is particularly common with acute MI, and it may be a sign of reperfusion after the use of thrombolytic agents. The arrhythmia is generally

---

*Consult the Bibliography and other more specialized sources for detailed discussions of ICD technology and other nonpharmacologic modalities for treating refractory ventricular arrhythmias (i.e., surgery, antitachycardia pacemakers, and catheter ablation techniques).

Classification of Ventricular Tachycardia

Duration

Nonsustained (lasting three beats to 30 seconds)
Sustained (lasting 30 seconds or more, or somewhat shorter runs if associated with symptoms of syncope or near-syncope)

Morphology

Monomorphic
Polymorphic
  With long QT(U) syndrome: torsade de pointes
  Without long QT(U) syndrome: for example, polymorphic ventricular tachycardia with acute ischemia

---

short lived, lasting minutes or less, and usually requires no specific therapy.

In many cases (see Fig. 14.15), AIVR appears to be a benign "escape" rhythm that competes with the underlying sinus mechanism. When the sinus rate slows, AIVR appears; when the sinus rate speeds up, the arrhythmia disappears. In other cases (see Fig. 14.16), AIVR is initiated by premature beats rather than escape beats. This latter type is more likely to be associated with actual VT.

Fig. 14.16 Accelerated idioventricular rhythm *(AIVR)* and nonsustained polymorphic ventricular tachycardia *(VT)* occurring together. Notice the "VPB on T" beats that initiate both the AIVR and the VT episodes.

Torsade de Pointes: A Specific Form of Polymorphic Ventricular Tachycardia

A distinct type of polymorphic VT is called *torsade de pointes* (a French term meaning "twisting of the points"). Figs. 14.17 and 14.18 show examples of this tachycardia. Notice how the direction of the QRS complexes appears to rotate cyclically, pointing downward for several beats and then twisting and pointing upward in the same lead.

Torsade de pointes is important because of its diagnostic and therapeutic implications. As shown in Fig. 14.17, *torsade de pointes occurs in the setting of delayed ventricular repolarization, evidenced by prolongation of the QT intervals or the presence of prominent U waves*. It is often initiated by a VPB that occurs near or on the T or U wave of the preceding beat. Reported causes include the following (also see Chapter 22):

- Drugs, particularly quinidine (see Chapter 10) and related antiarrhythmic agents (disopyramide and procainamide), sotalol, amiodarone (less commonly), psychotropic agents (phenothiazines and tricyclic antidepressants), terfenadine, and others
- Electrolyte imbalances, including hypokalemia, hypomagnesemia, and less commonly, hypocalcemia, which prolong repolarization
- Miscellaneous factors such as severe bradyarrhythmias, liquid protein diets, and hereditary long-QT syndromes

Recognition of torsade de pointes is critical because this ventricular tachycardia is often caused by drugs conventionally recommended for the treatment of arrhythmias. Therefore the therapy of torsade de pointes must include removing or correcting causative factors such as drug toxicity, electrolyte imbalance, or underlying bradycardia. In emergency settings a temporary pacemaker may be inserted to accomplish "overdrive" suppression of the arrhythmia by increasing the underlying heart rate and thereby decreasing ventricular repolarization time. Intravenous magnesium sulfate has proved highly useful for suppressing this arrhythmia. Drug therapy with isoproterenol or bretylium has been used in selected cases. Sustained episodes of torsade de pointes require attempted cardioversion. However, the arrhythmia usually recurs unless causative factors are corrected.*

Polymorphic VT may also occur without QT prolongation (see Fig. 14.16), for example, in the setting of acute myocardial ischemia.

Ventricular Fibrillation

With VF (see Figs. 14.13 and 14.14), the ventricles do not beat in any coordinated fashion but instead fibrillate or quiver asynchronously and ineffectively. No cardiac output occurs, and the patient becomes unconscious immediately. VF is one of the three major ECG patterns seen with cardiac arrest. The other two are *bradyasystolic patterns* and *electromechanical dissociation* (see Chapter 17).

---

*Consult texts cited in the Bibliography for further discussions of torsade de pointes.

Torsade de Pointes: Nonsustained

Fig. 14.17 Notice the shifting polarity and amplitude of the QRS complexes during an episode of nonsustained torsade de pointes. QT(U) prolongation (0.52 second) is also present in the normal sinus beats.

Torsade de Pointes: Sustained

Monitor lead

Fig. 14.18 Classic pattern of the sustained torsade de pointes type of ventricular tachycardia. Notice the pattern of beats in which the QRS axis appears to rotate or turn in a systematic way. Fig. 14.17 shows a short, nonsustained run of the same arrhythmia, which occurs in the setting of QT(U) prolongation.

The ECG in VF shows characteristic fibrillatory waves with an irregular pattern that may be either coarse or fine (see Fig. 14.13).

VF requires immediate defibrillation with an unsynchronized DC shock. Patients who have just been resuscitated from an episode of VF are generally given an immediate dose of an intravenous antiarrhythmic drug in an attempt to suppress further ventricular ectopy.

This lethal tachyarrhythmia can occur in patients with heart disease of any type. It may be preceded by a warning arrhythmia (e.g., VPBs or VT), or it may occur spontaneously. VF is the most common cause of *sudden cardiac death* (see Chapter 17) in patients with acute MI, although it may also occur in normal hearts, sometimes because of drugs (e.g., epinephrine).

Review

Ventricular premature beats (VPBs) may occur normally or with organic heart disease. VPBs have the following characteristics:

1. They are premature, occurring before the next normal beat is expected.
2. They have an aberrant shape. The QRS complex is abnormally wide, usually 0.12 second or more in duration, and the T wave and QRS complex usually point in opposite directions.

VPBs may occur with varying frequency. Two in a row are called a *couplet.* Three or more in a row constitute *ventricular tachycardia (VT).* When a VPB occurs regularly after each normal beat, the grouping is called *ventricular bigeminy.* When the rhythm is two normal beats followed by a VPB, this grouping is termed *ventricular trigeminy.*

A VPB is often followed by a compensatory pause before the next beat. *Uniform* VPBs have the same shape in a single lead. *Multiform* VPBs have different shapes in the same lead.

A VPB occurring simultaneously with the apex of the T wave of the preceding beat is called an *R on T phenomenon.* It may be the precursor of VT or ventricular fibrillation (VF), particularly in the setting of acute myocardial infarction or long QT syndromes.

VT is a run of three or more VPBs. Short runs of VT are called *nonsustained.* In *sustained* VT, episodes last more than 30 seconds and may lead to syncope or even cardiac arrest. VT may be classified as *monomorphic* or *polymorphic. Torsade de pointes* is a particular type of polymorphic VT associated with prolonged repolarization syndromes such as long QT(U) syndrome.

Accelerated idioventricular rhythm (AIVR) is a ventricular arrhythmia that resembles a slow VT with a rate between 50 and 100 beats/min. It is commonly seen with MI and is usually self-limited.

Torsade de pointes is a form of VT in which the QRS complexes in the same lead appear to twist periodically and turn in the opposite direction. It is generally seen in the setting of delayed ventricular repolarization (increased QT interval or prominent U waves) caused by drugs (quinidine), electrolyte abnormalities (hypokalemia, hypomagnesemia), or other factors.

VF occurs when the ventricles stop beating and, instead, fibrillate or twitch in an ineffective fashion. It is one of the three major ECG patterns seen with cardiac arrest; the other two are *brady-asystole* and *electromechanical dissociation* (see Chapter 17).

Questions

1. What is the arrhythmia shown below?

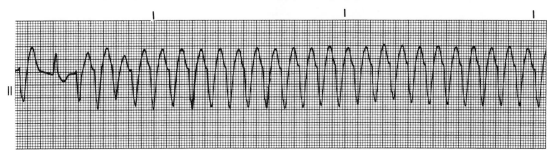

2. Which arrhythmia does this rhythm strip show?

Monitor lead

1 sec

3. Name three potentially treatable causes of ventricular premature beats.
4. What is the rhythm here?

15

Atrioventricular Heart Block

*H*eart block is the general term for atrioventricular (AV) conduction disturbances. Normally the AV junction (node) acts as a bridge between the atria and ventricles. As mentioned in Chapter 2, the PR interval is primarily a measure of the lag in AV conduction between initial stimulation of the atria and initial stimulation of the ventricles. The normal PR interval is between 0.12 and 0.2 second.

Heart block occurs when transmission through the AV junction is impaired either transiently or permanently (Table 15.1). The mildest form is called *first-degree heart block.* However, the term *first-degree AV block* is actually a misnomer because the impulse is not blocked but delayed. Therefore a preferable term is *prolonged PR interval.* With first-degree heart block the PR interval is uniformly prolonged above 0.2 second. *Second-degree heart block* is an intermediate grade of AV conduction disturbance in which impulse transmission between the atria and ventricles fails *intermittently.* The most extreme form is *third-degree* or *complete heart block.* In this case the AV junction does not conduct any stimuli between the atria and ventricles. These three degrees of heart block are described in the present chapter, along with the related topic *AV dissociation.*

Prolonged PR Interval (First-Degree Heart Block)

With first-degree heart block the PR interval is prolonged above 0.2 second and is constant from beat to beat (Fig. 15.1). A prolonged PR interval does not produce symptoms or significant change in cardiac function. The PR interval may become prolonged for many reasons. Most factors that produce PR prolongation can also produce second- and third-degree block. For example, digitalis, which has a vagal effect on the AV junction, can produce any degree of heart block. Other drugs such as amiodarone, beta blockers, and calcium channel blockers (e.g., verapamil and diltiazem) can also severely depress AV conduction.

Patients with ischemic heart disease may have heart block of any degree. This may occur with chronic myocardial ischemia over a long time or with acute myocardial infarction (MI). Varying degrees of heart block are particularly common with inferior wall infarction because the right coronary artery, which generally supplies the inferior wall of the heart, also usually supplies the AV junction. In addition, acute inferior MI is often associated with increased vagal tone. Heart block during inferior wall infarction tends to be transient.

Hyperkalemia may cause prolonged AV conduction. Other signs of hyperkalemia include peaking of the T waves and widening of the QRS complexes (see Chapter 10). Prolonged PR intervals may also occur with acute rheumatic fever. Not uncommonly, mild PR interval prolongation is seen as a normal variant, especially with physiologic sinus bradycardia during rest or sleep.

Second-Degree AV Block

Second-degree AV block is somewhat more complicated because it has two types: *Mobitz type I*

First-Degree AV Block

PR = 0.34 second

Fig. 15.1 With first-degree atrioventricular block the PR interval is uniformly prolonged above 0.2 second with each beat.

block (also called *Wenckebach block*) and *Mobitz type II block.*

MOBITZ TYPE I (WENCKEBACH) AV BLOCK

With the Mobitz type I or Wenckebach pattern, each stimulus from the atria to the ventricles appears to have a more difficult time passing through the AV junction. Finally the stimulus is not conducted at all. This *blocked beat* is followed by relative recovery of the AV junction, and the whole cycle starts again.

The characteristic ECG picture of Wenckebach block is progressive lengthening of the PR interval from beat to beat until a beat is "dropped." The dropped beat is a P wave that is not followed by a QRS complex, indicating failure of the AV junction to conduct the stimulus from the atria to the ventricles. Furthermore, the PR interval following the nonconducted P wave is shorter than the PR interval of the beat just before the nonconducted P wave. Fig. 15.2 diagrammatically depicts the Wenckebach phenomenon, and Fig. 15.3 shows an actual example of this pattern. The number of P waves occurring before a QRS complex is dropped may vary. In many cases just two or three P waves are seen. What characterizes the Wenckebach pattern is the general sequence of a progressive lengthening of the PR interval followed by a nonconducted P wave.

As you can see from the examples, the Wenckebach cycle also produces a distinct clustering of QRS complexes separated by a pause that results from the dropped beat. Any time you encounter an ECG with this type of *group beating,* you should

Table 15.1 Classification of AV Heart Blocks

Degree	AV conduction pattern
First-degree block	Uniformly prolonged PR interval
Second-degree block*	Intermittent conduction failure* Mobitz type I (Wenckebach): progressive PR prolongation Mobitz type II: sudden conduction failure
Third-degree block	No atrioventricular conduction

*Two special types are sometimes designated: 2:1 atrioventricular block and advanced atrioventricular block (3:1, 4:1, etc.)

suspect a Wenckebach block and look for the diagnostic pattern of lengthening PR intervals.

Clinically, patients with the Wenckebach type of AV block are usually without symptoms unless the ventricular rate is very slow. The pulse rate is irregular.

Common causes of Wenckebach block include ischemic heart disease and drugs such as digitalis, beta blockers, and calcium channel blockers (diltiazem and verapamil). Wenckebach block is not uncommon with acute inferior wall MI. In such cases it is usually transient and generally does not require any treatment except observation. Occasionally these patients may progress into complete heart block. Of note, a physiologic increase in vagal tone may cause Wenckebach AV block in athletes at rest.

Mobitz Type I (Wenckebach) Second-Degree AV Block

Fig. 15.2 The PR interval lengthens progressively with successive beats until one P wave is not conducted at all. Then the cycle repeats itself. Notice that the PR interval following the nonconducted P wave is shorter than the PR interval of the beat just before it.

Mobitz Type I (Wenckebach) Second-Degree AV Block

Fig. 15.3 Notice the progressive increase in PR intervals, with the third P wave in each sequence not followed by a QRS complex. Mobitz type I (Wenckebach) block produces a characteristically syncopated rhythm with grouping of the QRS complexes (group beating).

MOBITZ TYPE II AV BLOCK

Mobitz type II AV block is a rarer and more serious form of second-degree heart block. Its characteristic feature is the sudden appearance of a nonconducted sinus P wave without the progressive prolongation of PR intervals seen in Mobitz type I (Wenckebach) AV block.*

Mobitz type II block is generally a sign of severe conduction system disease involving regions below the AV node (i.e., His-Purkinje system). Because Mobitz type II block often progresses into complete heart block, cardiologists generally consider it an indication for a pacemaker. Unlike Wenckebach AV block, Mobitz type II block is *not* seen with digitalis excess or inferior wall MI. However, Mobitz type II block may be seen with anterior wall MI, and these patients often progress into complete heart block. Therefore

---

*For clarification of a point of common confusion, it should be noted that 2:1 AV block per se does not necessarily indicate a Mobitz type II block. Not uncommonly, 2:1 AV block is due to a type I mechanism in which the block in the AV node occurs after every other P wave. In such cases a careful search of a long rhythm strip often reveals 3:2, 4:3, etc. types of Wenckebach block in addition to the 2:1 periods. Furthermore, in most (but not all) cases of Wenckebach AV block the QRS complex is of normal duration. By contrast, when 2:1 block is due to a type II mechanism, the His-Purkinje system (not just the AV node) is involved and the QRS duration is often prolonged. Thus 2:1 block with a narrow QRS complex most likely represents a type I mechanism. However, 2:1 block with a wide QRS complex may be due to either mechanism. Definitive assessment in any case of 2:1 block may require an intracardiac electrophysiologic study. Therefore pure 2:1 block can be labeled as such without specifying a type I or type II mechanism.

Fig. 15.4 Lead II recorded during a Holter monitor ECG in a patient with intermittent light-headedness. The recording shows sinus rhythm with 2:1 block alternating with 3:1 block (i.e., two consecutive nonconducted P waves followed by a conducted one). The term *advanced second-degree atrioventricular block* is applied when the ECG shows two or more nonconducted P waves in a row.

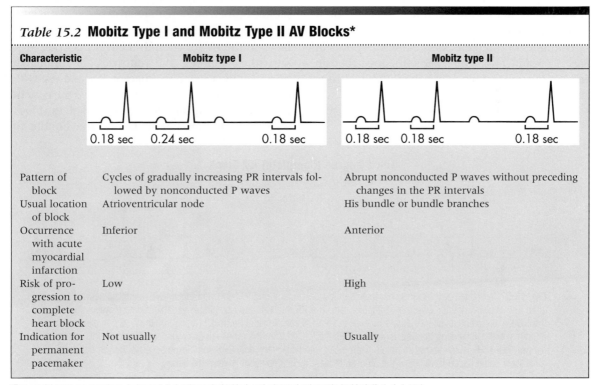

Table 15.2 **Mobitz Type I and Mobitz Type II AV Blocks***

Characteristic	Mobitz type I	Mobitz type II
	0.18 sec 0.24 sec 0.18 sec	0.18 sec 0.18 sec 0.18 sec
Pattern of block	Cycles of gradually increasing PR intervals followed by nonconducted P waves	Abrupt nonconducted P waves without preceding changes in the PR intervals
Usual location of block	Atrioventricular node	His bundle or bundle branches
Occurrence with acute myocardial infarction	Inferior	Anterior
Risk of progression to complete heart block	Low	High
Indication for permanent pacemaker	Not usually	Usually

*Two special types are sometimes designated: 2:1 atrioventricular block and advanced atrioventricular block (3:1, 4:1, etc.)

cardiologists generally treat patients with anterior wall MI and Mobitz type II AV block by inserting a pacemaker.

Mobitz I and Mobitz II AV blocks are compared in Table 15.2.

The term *advanced second-degree AV block* refers to the ECG finding of two or more consecutive nonconducted P waves (Fig. 15.4). For example, with sinus rhythm and 3:1 block, every third P wave is conducted; with 4:1 block, every fourth P wave is conducted, and so forth. Unless advanced second-degree AV block has a reversible cause (e.g., drug toxicity or hyperkalemia), a permanent pacemaker is usually required.

Third-Degree (Complete) Heart Block

First- and second-degree heart blocks are examples of *incomplete* block because the AV junction conducts at least some stimuli to the ventricles. With complete heart block, no stimuli are transmitted from the atria to the ventricles. Instead, the atria and ventricles are paced independently. The atria generally continue to be paced by the sinus node, or sinoatrial (SA), node. The ventricles, however, are paced by an escape pacemaker located somewhere below the point of block in the AV junction. The resting ventricular rate with complete heart block may be lower than 30 beats/min or as high as 50 to 60 beats/min. The atrial rate is generally faster than the ventricular rate.

Examples of complete heart block are shown in Figs. 15.5 and 15.6. The ECG with sinus rhythm and complete heart block has the following three characteristics:

- P waves are present, with a regular atrial rate faster than the ventricular rate.

- QRS complexes are present, with a slow (usually fixed) ventricular rate.
- The P waves bear no relation to the QRS complexes, and the PR intervals are completely variable because the atria and ventricles are electrically disconnected.

Complete heart block may also occur in patients whose basic atrial rhythm is flutter or fibrillation. In these cases the ventricular rate is very slow and almost completely regular (see Fig. 13.8).

With complete heart block the QRS complexes may be either of normal width (Fig. 15.5) or abnormally wide (Fig. 15.6) with the appearance of a bundle branch block pattern. The width of the QRS complexes depends in part on the location of the block in the AV junction. If the block is in the first part (the AV node), the ventricles are stimulated normally by a junctional pacemaker and the QRS complexes are narrow (Fig. 15.5) unless the patient has an underlying bundle branch block. If the block is within, or particularly below, the bundle of

Third-Degree (Complete) AV Block

Fig. 15.5 Complete heart block is characterized by independent atrial *(P)* and ventricular (QRS complex) activity. The atrial rate is always faster than the ventricular rate. The PR intervals are completely variable. Some P waves fall on the T wave, distorting its shape. Others may fall in the QRS complex and be "lost." Notice that the QRS complexes are of normal width, indicating that the ventricles are being paced from the atrioventricular junction. Compare this example with Fig. 15.6, which shows complete heart block with wide, very slow QRS complexes because the ventricles are most likely being paced from below the atrioventricular junction (idioventricular pacemaker).

Fig. 15.6 This example of complete heart block shows a very slow idioventricular rhythm and a faster independent atrial (sinus) rhythm (*P,* P wave).

His, the ventricles are paced by an *idioventricular pacemaker,** producing wide QRS complexes (Fig. 15.6). As a general clinical rule, complete heart block with wide QRS complexes tends to be less stable than complete heart block with narrow QRS complexes because the ventricular escape pacemaker is usually slower and less consistent.

Complete heart block can occur for a number of reasons. It is most commonly seen in older patients who have chronic degenerative changes (sclerosis or fibrosis) in their conduction systems *not* related to MI. Digitalis intoxication, which can cause second-degree heart block, may also lead to complete heart block (see Chapter 16). Varying degrees of AV block, including some cases of complete block, have been reported with Lyme disease. Complete heart block may occur abruptly after open-heart surgery, particularly with aortic valve replacement. Complete heart block occurring with bacterial endocarditis is an ominous finding that suggests an abscess involving the conduction system.

Complete heart block may also be seen acutely as a complication of MI. The course and therapy of complete heart block with MI depend to a large extent on whether the infarct is anterior or inferior. Transient AV conduction disturbances are commonly seen with acute inferior wall MI because of the common blood supply to the AV junction and inferior wall (via the right coronary artery). Occlusion of the right coronary artery with inferior MI also often leads to temporary ischemia of the AV node, sometimes resulting in complete heart block. (In addition, acute inferior MI may cause an increase in vagal tone.) Complete heart block occurring with inferior wall MI is often a transient and reversible complication that does not usually require a temporary pacemaker unless the patient is hypotensive or is having episodes of tachyarrhythmia.

With acute anterior MI and complete heart block, the situation is more serious. Patients with anterior wall infarcts and complete heart block generally have extensive myocardial damage. The idioventricular escape rhythm that develops is usually slow and unstable. Therefore if complete heart block occurs with an acute anterior MI, cardiologists insert a temporary pacemaker (and subsequently a permanent one).

Regardless of its cause, complete heart block is a serious and potentially life-threatening arrhythmia. If the ventricular rate becomes too slow, the cardiac output drops and the patient may faint. Fainting spells associated with complete heart block (or other types of bradycardia) are referred to as *Stokes-Adams attacks.* In some patients, complete heart block is a chronic and persistent finding. In others the block may occur transiently and may be recognized only with more prolonged monitoring.

Bifascicular Block, Trifascicular Block, and Complete Heart Block

Cardiologists have been interested in developing criteria to predict which patients with acute MI (particularly anterior wall infarcts) will develop life-threatening complete heart block. Current information suggests that certain high-risk patients can be identified, although precise predictions are not possible. Specifically, patients with acute anterior wall MI and complete heart block often have other conduction disturbances before the onset of complete heart block. These conduction disturbances are referred to as *bifascicular blocks.*

Recall from Chapter 7 that the ventricular conduction system is *trifascicular,* consisting of the right bundle branch and the left bundle branch, the latter further dividing into left anterior and left posterior fascicles. Blockage of just the left anterior fascicle produces left anterior fascicular block (hemiblock) with left axis deviation (LAD). Blockage of just the left posterior fascicle produces left posterior fascicular block (hemiblock) with right axis deviation (RAD). Bifascicular block indicates blockage of any two of the three fascicles. For example, right bundle branch block (RBBB) with left anterior hemiblock produces an RBBB pattern with marked LAD (see Figs. 8.20 and 15.7); RBBB with left posterior hemiblock produces an RBBB pattern with RAD (provided other causes of RAD, especially right ventricular hypertrophy and lateral MI, are excluded). Similarly, a complete LBBB

---

*An idioventricular pacemaker may be located in the His-Purkinje system or the ventricular myocardium.

may indicate blockage of both the anterior and posterior fascicles.

Bifascicular blocks are potentially significant because they make ventricular conduction dependent on the single remaining fascicle. Additional damage to this third remaining fascicle may completely block AV conduction, producing complete heart block *(trifascicular block)*. Therefore the acute development of new bifascicular block (especially with a prolonged PR interval) during an acute anterior wall MI is a warning signal of possible impending complete heart block.

An important distinction must be made between *acute* bifascicular blocks occurring with anterior wall MI (see Fig. 8.20) and *chronic* bifascicular blocks (see Fig. 15.7). Many people with no symptoms at all may have ECGs resembling the one in Fig. 15.7. Patients with chronic bifascicu-

Bifascicular Block (Right Bundle Branch Block with Left Anterior Hemiblock)

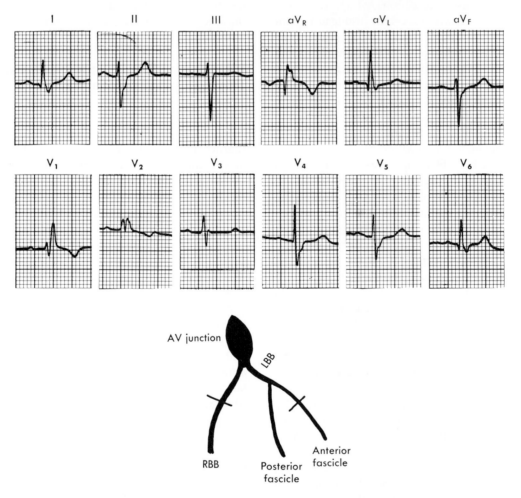

Fig. 15.7 Notice that the chest leads show the typical right bundle branch block pattern (rSR′ in lead V₁ and qRS in lead V₆). The extremity leads show marked left axis deviation (mean QRS axis about −60 degrees), consistent with left anterior hemiblock. Thus a bifascicular block involving the right bundle branch *(RBB)* and the anterior fascicle of the left bundle branch *(LBB)* system is present (as shown in the diagram) *(AV,* atrioventricular).

lar block do not generally require a permanent pacemaker unless they develop second- or third-degree AV block. The risk of complete heart block in patients with *chronic* bifascicular block seems to be quite low. By contrast, patients with acute anterior MI in whom bifascicular block suddenly occurs have a poor prognosis because of underlying extensive myocardial necrosis, and they are also at higher risk of developing complete heart block.

AV Dissociation

Cardiologists use the term *AV dissociation* in two related though not identical ways. This classification continues to cause considerable (and understandable) confusion among students and clinicians.

AV dissociation is widely used as a *general* term for any arrhythmia in which the atria and ventricles are controlled by independent pacemakers. The definition includes complete heart block, as well as some instances of ventricular tachycardia in which the atria remain in sinus rhythm (see Chapter 18).

AV dissociation is also used as a more *specific* term to describe a particular family of arrhythmias that are often mistaken for complete heart block. With this type of AV dissociation the SA node and AV junction appear to be "out of synch"; thus the SA node loses its normal control of the ventricular rate. As a result the atria and ventricles are paced independently—the atria from the SA node, the ventricles from the AV junction. This is similar to what occurs with complete heart block. *However, with AV dissociation the ventricular rate is the same as or slightly faster than the atrial rate.* When the atrial and ventricular rates are almost the same, the term *isorhythmic AV dissociation* is used.

The critical difference between AV dissociation (resulting from "desynchronization" of the SA and AV nodes) and actual complete heart block (resulting from conduction failure) is as follows: with AV dissociation (e.g., isorhythmic) a properly timed P wave can be conducted through the AV node whereas with complete heart block no P wave reaches the ventricles.

AV dissociation (Fig. 15.8) therefore can be regarded as a "competition" between the SA node and the AV node for control of the heartbeat. It may occur either when the SA node slows down (e.g., because of the effects of beta blockers or calcium channel blockers or with increased vagal tone) or when the AV node is accelerated (e.g., by ischemia or digitalis toxicity). Not uncommonly, isorhythmic AV dissociation is seen in healthy young individuals, particularly when they are sleeping.

Fig. 15.8 presents an example of isorhythmic AV dissociation. Notice the P waves with a variable PR interval because the ventricular (QRS) rate is nearly the same as the atrial rate. At times the P waves may merge with the QRS complexes and become imperceptible for several beats. If the sinus rate speeds up sufficiently (or the AV junctional rate slows), the stimulus may be able to penetrate the AV junction, reestablishing sinus rhythm.

Isorhythmic AV Dissociation

Fig. 15.8 This type of atrioventricular (AV) dissociation is characterized by transient desynchronization of the sino-atrial and AV node pacemakers such that they beat at nearly the same rate. Because they are "out of synch" with each other, the *P* waves (representing the sinus node pacemaker) appear to slide in and out of the QRS (representing the AV junction pacemaker). This type of AV dissociation must be distinguished from actual complete AV block (see Figs. 15.5 and 15.6).

Review

Three types of atrioventricular (AV) heart block may occur:

1. With PR interval prolongation, or *first-degree block,* the PR interval uniformly is prolonged beyond 0.2 second.
2. *Second-degree* heart block has two major types, with two special subtypes sometimes designated:
   a. In *Mobitz type I (Wenckebach) block,* the PR interval is increasingly prolonged until a P wave is blocked and not followed by a QRS complex; this produces a distinctive clustering of QRS complexes separated by a pause resulting from the dropped beat (known as *group beating*).
   b. In *Mobitz type II block,* a nonconducted sinus P wave appears suddenly without prolongation of the preceding PR interval; also the PR interval following the nonconducted P wave is the same as the one before it.
   c. Two special subtypes have been designated: *2:1 AV block,* which may be due to a type I or type II mechanism, and *advanced second-degree atrioventricular block,* in which two or more nonconducted P waves are present (i.e., 3:1 or 4:1 block).
3. *Third-degree (complete) block* shows the following:
   a. Atria and ventricles that beat independently because stimuli cannot pass through the AV junction
   b. An atrial rate that is almost always faster than the ventricular rate
   c. A PR interval that is constantly changing

Complete heart block with acute anterior wall myocardial infarction (MI) is sometimes preceded by the sudden appearance of *bifascicular block* (right bundle branch block with left anterior or posterior fascicular block or a new complete left bundle branch block). However, patients with *chronic* bifascicular block who have no symptoms usually do not require any special therapy.

The significance of complete heart block with acute MI depends on the location of the infarct. Complete heart block occurring with acute inferior wall MI is usually transient and can sometimes be managed without a pacemaker. By contrast, complete heart block with acute anterior wall MI is usually associated with a very poor prognosis and requires a pacemaker.

Complete heart block must be distinguished from other forms of *AV dissociation.* With *isorhythmic* AV dissociation the atria and ventricles beat independently; however, the ventricular rate is about the same as the atrial rate. AV dissociation of this type is a minor, usually transient arrhythmia.

Questions

1. The rhythm strip below shows sinus rhythm with which of the following?
   a. Wenckebach-type second-degree atrioventricular (AV) block
   b. Complete heart block
   c. 3:1 AV block
   d. AV dissociation
   e. Blocked premature atrial beats

2. Based on the rhythm strip below, answer the following questions:
   a. What is the approximate atrial (P wave) rate?
   b. What is the approximate ventricular (QRS) rate?
   c. Is the PR interval constant?
   d. What is the ECG abnormality shown?

16

Digitalis Toxicity

*T*his chapter focuses on the arrhythmias and conduction disturbances caused by digitalis intoxication. This subject is included in an introductory textbook for several reasons. The most important is that digitalis is a frequently prescribed drug and digitalis toxicity remains an important clinical problem. Furthermore, digitalis toxicity can cause fatal arrhythmias. Therefore all clinicians should strive to recognize digitalis toxicity early. Finally, because digitalis toxicity can produce a wide variety of arrhythmias and all degrees of heart block, this topic provides a convenient review of material presented in previous chapters.

Clinical Background

Digitalis refers to a class of cardiac drugs (glycosides) with specific effects on the mechanical and electrical function of the heart. The most commonly used digitalis preparation is digoxin.

Digitalis is used in clinical practice for two major reasons. First, in selected patients with dilated hearts and congestive heart failure (CHF) it increases the strength of myocardial contractions. This is its *mechanical* action. Second, it affects the conductivity of certain heart tissues. This is its *electrical* action. Thus digitalis is useful for treating selected arrhythmias. Its antiarrhythmic action results primarily from its slowing of conduction through the atrioventricular (AV) junction (node) as the result of an increase in vagal tone. Consequently, digitalis is used for controlling the ventricular response in atrial fibrillation (AF) and atrial flutter, which are characterized by the ex-

cessive transmission of stimuli from the atria to the ventricles through the AV junction. It also is used to treat certain reentrant types of paroxysmal supraventricular tachycardia (PSVT).*

Unfortunately, although digitalis has wide use in the treatment of heart failure and selected arrhythmias, it also has a relatively low margin of safety. The difference between therapeutic and toxic concentrations is very narrow.

Signs of Digitalis Toxicity

Digitalis toxicity can produce general systemic symptoms as well as specific cardiac arrhythmias and conduction disturbances. Common extracardiac symptoms include weakness, anorexia, nausea, and vomiting. Visual effects (altered color perception) and mental changes may occur. This section of the chapter concentrates on the arrhythmias and conduction disturbances produced by digitalis excess.

As a general clinical rule *virtually any arrhythmia and all degrees of AV heart block can be produced by digitalis intoxication.* Of all the arrhythmias discussed in this book, AF and atrial flutter with a rapid ventricular response are the *least* likely to be caused by digitalis toxicity. However, a number of

---

*The basic mechanisms involved in digitalis-related arrhythmias are complex and incompletely understood. Bradyarrhythmias may be due to excessive increases in vagal tone caused by digitalis. Increased automaticity and tachycardias may be due to the effects of toxic doses of digitalis on the sympathetic nervous system. The automaticity of cardiac cells in the atria, AV junction, and ventricles may also be directly enhanced by digitalis, leading to some of the arrhythmias described in this chapter.

other arrhythmias and conduction disturbances are commonly seen with digitalis toxicity (box).

VENTRICULAR ARRHYTHMIAS

Ventricular premature beats (VPBs) are often the first sign of digitalis toxicity. Isolated VPBs may occur at first. Ventricular bigeminy (Fig. 16.1), with each normal beat followed by a VPB, is common. Ventricular tachycardia (VT) and fatal ventricular fibrillation (VF) may occur if digitalis toxicity is not recognized and treated (see Chapter 17).

BIDIRECTIONAL VENTRICULAR TACHYCARDIA

Bidirectional VT (Fig. 16.2) is a special type of VT in which each successive beat in any lead alternates in direction. This distinctive tachyarrhythmia should always raise the question of digitalis intoxication.

AV JUNCTIONAL (NODAL) RHYTHMS

AV junctional rhythms are frequently a sign of digitalis toxicity.* Most AV junctional rhythms re-

---

*Two classes of junctional (nodal) rhythms may occur: (1) a typical junctional escape rhythm with a rate of 60 beats/min or less and (2) an accelerated junctional rhythm (also called nonparoxysmal junctional tachycardia) at a rate of about 60 to 130 beats/min.

sulting from excessive digitalis have a rate of less than 130 beats/min.

SINUS BRADYCARDIA AND SINOATRIAL BLOCK

Sinus bradycardia may be one of the earliest signs of digitalis excess. Sinoatrial (SA) block with sinus arrest may also occur.

Common Arrhythmias and Conduction Disturbances Caused by Digitalis Toxicity

Bradycardias

Sinus bradycardia (including sinoatrial block)
Junctional (nodal) escape rhythms*
Atrioventricular (AV) heart block, including Mobitz type I (Wenckebach) AV block and complete heart block*

Tachycardias

Accelerated or junctional rhythm such as nonparoxysmal or junctional tachycardia*
Atrial tachycardia with block
Ventricular ectopy, including ventricular premature beats, monomorphic ventricular tachycardia, bidirectional ventricular tachycardia, and ventricular fibrillation

---

*These arrhythmias and conduction disturbances may occur with underlying atrial fibrillation leading to slow or regularized ventricular response. Atrioventricular dissociation without complete heart block may also occur.

Fig. 16.1 Ventricular bigeminy caused by digitalis toxicity. Ventricular ectopy is one of the most common signs of digitalis toxicity. **A,** The underlying rhythm is atrial fibrillation. **B,** Each normal QRS complex is followed by a ventricular premature beat.

Bidirectional Tachycardia

Fig. 16.2 This digitalis-toxic arrhythmia is a special type of ventricular tachycardia with QRS complexes that alternate in direction from beat to beat. No P waves are present.

Atrial Tachycardia with Block

Fig. 16.3 This rhythm strip shows atrial tachycardia (about 200 beats/min) with 2:1 block, producing a ventricular rate of about 100 beats/min.

ATRIAL TACHYCARDIA WITH AV BLOCK

Atrial tachycardia (AT) with AV block is another tachyarrhythmia that has not been discussed in earlier chapters (an example appears in Fig. 16.3). This arrhythmia is usually characterized by regular, rapid P waves occurring at a rate between 150 and 250 beats/min and, because of the AV block, a slower ventricular rate. Not uncommonly, 2:1 AV block is present so that the ventricular rate is half the atrial rate. Mobitz type I (Wenckebach) AV block is also common. Digitalis toxicity is an important, but not the only, cause of these arrhythmias. Superficially, AT with block may resemble atrial flutter; however, in AT with block the baseline between P waves is isoelectric. Furthermore, when atrial flutter is present, the atrial rate is faster (usually 250 to 350 beats/min).

AV HEART BLOCK AND AV DISSOCIATION

Because digitalis slows conduction through the AV junction, it is not surprising that toxic doses can result in any degree of AV heart block.

First-Degree Block

With first-degree AV block, PR intervals are uniformly prolonged more than 0.2 second. Some

Fig. 16.4 Atrial fibrillation with an excessively slow ventricular rate because of digitalis toxicity. Atrial fibrillation with a rapid ventricular rate is rarely caused by digitalis toxicity. However, in patients with underlying atrial fibrillation, digitalis toxicity is often manifested by excessive slowing or regularization of the QRS rate.

degree of PR lengthening may be expected with digitalis therapy. More marked widening of the PR interval suggests early digitalis toxicity.

Second-Degree Block

With higher doses of digitalis, PR prolongation may progress to second-degree block of the Mobitz type I (Wenckebach) variety.

Complete Heart Block

Third-degree, or complete, heart block may also occur with digitalis toxicity.

Digitalis toxicity may also cause other types of AV dissociation (see Chapter 15).

ATRIAL FIBRILLATION OR FLUTTER WITH SLOW VENTRICULAR RATE

Rarely, digitalis causes AF and atrial flutter with a rapid ventricular response. In such cases the toxicity is often shown by marked slowing of the ventricular rate to less than 50 beats/min (Fig. 16.4) and/or the appearance of VPBs. In some cases the earliest sign of digitalis toxicity in a patient with AF may be a subtle *regularization* of the ventricular rate.

In summary, digitalis toxicity causes a number of important arrhythmias and conduction disturbances. Therefore because of the frequency and potential lethality of digitalis toxicity you should suspect this problem in any patient taking a digi-

---

Predisposing Factors for Digitalis Toxicity

Hypokalemia
Hypomagnesemia
Hypercalcemia
Hypoxemia
Chronic lung disease
Myocardial infarction
Old age
Renal insufficiency
Hypothyroidism
Hypertrophic cardiomyopathy (an inherited heart condition associated with excessive cardiac contractility)
Heart failure caused by amyloidosis
Wolff-Parkinson-White syndrome and atrial fibrillation

---

talis preparation who has an unexplained arrhythmia until you can prove otherwise.

Factors Predisposing to Digitalis Toxicity

A number of factors significantly increase the hazard of digitalis intoxication (box). For example, a low serum potassium concentration increases the likelihood of certain digitalis-induced arrhythmias, particularly ventricular ectopy and AT with block. Hypokalemia is not uncommon in patients who are taking digitalis because these patients frequently receive diuretics for the treatment of heart failure and edema. The serum potassium concentration must be checked periodically in any patient taking digitalis and in every patient suspected of having digitalis toxicity.

Hypomagnesemia occurs in a variety of settings, including alcoholism, intestinal malabsorption, and diuretic therapy. Hypercalcemia is seen with hyperparathyroidism and certain tumors, among other conditions. Both hypomagnesemia and hypercalcemia can be predisposing factors for digitalis toxicity.

Hypoxemia and chronic lung disease may also increase the risk of digitalis toxicity because they are associated with increased sympathetic tone.

Patients with acute myocardial infarction (MI) or ischemia appear to be more sensitive to digitalis.

Digoxin, the most widely used preparation of digitalis, is excreted primarily in the urine. Therefore any degree of renal insufficiency, as measured by increased blood urea nitrogen (BUN) and creatinine concentrations, requires a lower maintenance dose of digoxin. Thus elderly patients may be more susceptible to digitalis toxicity, in part because of decreased excretion of the drug.

Patients with hypothyroidism appear to be more sensitive to the effects of digitalis.

Even therapeutic levels of digoxin can be dangerous in certain patients. For example, digitalis may worsen the symptoms of patients with hypertrophic cardiomyopathy, an inherited heart condition associated with excessive cardiac contractility. Patients with heart failure due to amyloidosis are also extremely sensitive to digitalis. In patients with the Wolff-Parkinson-White syndrome and AF (see Chapter 18), digitalis may cause extremely rapid transmission of impulses down the atrioventricular bypass tract, leading to a potentially lethal tachycardia (see Fig. 18.10, *A*).

Treatment of Digitalis Toxicity

The first step in treatment is prevention. Before any patient is started on digoxin or a related drug, the indications should be carefully reviewed. Many patients continue to receive digoxin or related drugs for inappropriate reasons. The patient should have a baseline ECG, serum electrolytes, and BUN and creatinine measurements. Serum magnesium blood levels should also be considered, particularly if indicated by diuretic therapy, etc. Other considerations include the patient's age and pulmonary status, as well as whether the patient is having an acute MI. Early signs of digitalis toxicity (e.g., VPBs, sinus bradycardia, or increasing AV block) should be carefully checked. Furthermore, concomitant quinidine administration increases the digoxin level in patients who are taking both drugs. A similar effect occurs with other drugs, including verapamil, amiodarone, and propafenone.

Definitive treatment of digitalis toxicity depends on the particular arrhythmia. With minor arrhythmias (e.g., isolated VPBs, sinus bradycardia, prolonged PR interval, Wenckebach AV block or AV junctional rhythms), discontinuation of digitalis and careful observation are usually adequate. More serious arrhythmias (e.g., prolonged VT) may require suppression with an intravenous drug (lidocaine or procainamide). For tachycardias, potassium chloride should be given to raise the serum potassium level to well within normal limits. Patients with complete heart block from digitalis toxicity may require a temporary pacemaker while the effect of the digitalis dissipates, particularly if they have symptoms of syncope, hypotension, or CHF. In other cases, complete heart block can be managed conservatively while the digitalis wears off.

Occasionally patients present with a large overdose of digitalis taken inadvertently or in a suicide attempt. In such cases the serum digoxin level is markedly elevated, and severe bradyarrhythmia or tachyarrhythmias may develop. In addition, massive digitalis toxicity may cause life-threatening *hyperkalemia* because the drug blocks the cell membrane mechanism that pumps potassium into the cells in exchange for sodium. Patients with a potentially lethal overdose of digitalis can be treated with a special digitalis-binding antibody given intravenously (digoxin immune Fab [antigen-binding fragment; Digibind]). (Detailed accounts of the treatment of digitalis toxicity are given in selected texts cited in the Bibliography.)

Finally, *direct-current electrical cardioversion of arrhythmias in patients who have digitalis toxicity is extremely hazardous and may precipitate fatal ventricular tachycardia and fibrillation.* Therefore you should not electrically cardiovert any patient who has AT with block, AF, or atrial flutter and is suspected of having digitalis toxicity.

Serum Digoxin Levels

The concentration of digoxin in the serum can be measured by means of radioimmunoassay. Therapeutic concentrations range from about 0.5 to 2 ng/ml in most laboratories. Concentrations exceeding 2 ng/ml are associated with a high incidence of digitalis toxicity. In ordering a test of digoxin level in a patient, you must be aware that therapeutic levels do not rule out the possibility of digitalis toxicity. As previously mentioned, some patients are more sensitive to digitalis. In other patients, factors such as hypokalemia may produce digitalis toxicity despite a therapeutic serum level.* Although a "high" digoxin level does not necessarily indicate digitalis toxicity, these patients should be examined for early evidence of digitalis excess, including extracardiac symptoms (e.g., gastrointestinal symptoms) and all cardiac effects that have been discussed. (A spuriously high digoxin level may be obtained if blood is drawn within a few hours of the administration of digoxin.)

Digitalis Toxicity and Digitalis Effect

Digitalis toxicity, which refers to the arrhythmias and conduction disturbances produced by this drug, should not be confused with digitalis effect. *Digitalis effect* (see Fig. 10.1) refers to the distinct scooping of the ST-T complex seen in some patients who are taking digitalis. The presence of digitalis effect does not imply digitalis toxicity.

*The need for potentially toxic doses of digoxin to control the ventricular rate in AF has been obviated by the availability of other drugs (beta blockers and calcium channel blockers) and AV nodal ablation procedures (see Chapter 13).

Review

Digitalis toxicity can produce almost any arrhythmia and all degrees of AV heart block (see box on p. 189).

Atrial fibrillation or atrial flutter with a rapid ventricular response rarely occurs as a result of digitalis toxicity. Furthermore, digitalis toxicity does not produce bundle branch blocks.

Factors such as renal failure, hypokalemia, hypercalcemia, hypomagnesemia, hypoxemia, old age, and acute myocardial infarction are predisposing factors for digitalis toxicity. The concomitant administration of certain drugs (e.g., quinidine, verapamil, amiodarone, propafenone) also increases serum digoxin levels.

Digitalis toxicity should not be confused with digitalis effect. *Digitalis effect* refers to the shortening of the QT interval and scooping of the ST-T complex produced by *therapeutic* doses of digitalis.

Questions

1. Name three factors that can potentiate digitalis toxicity.

True or false (2 to 5):

2. Ventricular premature beats are a frequent manifestation of digitalis toxicity.
3. Atrial fibrillation with a rapid ventricular response is a common manifestation of digitalis toxicity.
4. Left bundle branch block may result from digitalis toxicity.
5. Mobitz type I (Wenckebach) atrioventricular block may be caused by digitalis toxicity.

17

Cardiac Arrest and Sudden Cardiac Death

*I*n the preceding chapters the major disorders of heart rhythm and atrioventricular (AV) conduction have been systematically discussed. Instead of considering entirely new ECG patterns, this chapter reviews some earlier topics, placing them in a special clinical perspective. The subject of this chapter is the recognition of life-threatening arrhythmias that cause cardiac arrest. By definition, *cardiac arrest occurs when the heart stops contracting effectively and ceases to pump blood.* The important and related topic of *sudden cardiac death* is also introduced.

Clinical Aspects of Cardiac Arrest

The patient in cardiac arrest loses consciousness within seconds and may even have a seizure as a result of inadequate blood flow to the brain. Irreversible brain damage usually occurs within 4 minutes and sometimes sooner. Furthermore, shortly after the heart stops pumping, spontaneous breathing also ceases *(cardiopulmonary arrest)*. Sometimes, when respirations stop first (primary respiratory arrest), cardiac activity stops shortly thereafter.

The diagnosis of cardiac arrest should be made clinically even before the patient is connected to an electrocardiograph. Cardiac arrest should be recognized immediately in any unconscious person who does not have palpable pulses. In this situation the clinician should examine patient quickly by trying to feel for pulses in the carotid arteries. The patient in cardiac arrest becomes cyanotic (bluish gray) from lack of oxygenated blood. No heart tones are audible with a stethoscope placed on the chest, and the blood pressure is, of course, unobtainable. The arms and legs become cool. If the brain becomes severely hypoxic, the pupils are fixed and dilated. Seizure activity may occur. However, *the absence of pulses in an unconscious person is the major diagnostic sign of cardiac arrest.*

When cardiac arrest is recognized, *cardiopulmonary resuscitation (CPR)* must be started without delay. In capsule form the initial treatment of any cardiac arrest consists of the following four *(A, B, C, D)* steps:

- Establish an *A*irway.
- *B*reathe for the patient, either by mouth-to-mouth or mouth-to-mask methods or by manually compressing a bag-valve device, forcing air into the patient's nose or mouth.
- Maintain *C*irculation by external cardiac compression.
- Begin *D*efinitive treatment with whatever intravenous or endotracheal drugs are needed, with electrical defibrillation, or with a temporary pacemaker when indicated.*

The details of CPR, including drug dosages, the use of defibrillators, and other matters, lie outside the scope of this book but are discussed in selected texts cited in the Bibliography. This chapter concentrates primarily on the particular ECG patterns

---

*While the above steps are being done by two or more rescuers, another rescuer can raise the patient's lower extremities to a vertical position and keep them elevated for 15 seconds. This may help return blood to the central circulation.

seen during cardiac arrest and the clinical implications of these patterns.

Initial treatment with ventilation and external cardiac compression should never be delayed while the patient in cardiac arrest is being connected to the electrocardiograph.

Basic ECG Patterns in Cardiac Arrest

The three basic ECG patterns seen with cardiac arrest were mentioned in earlier chapters. Cardiac arrest may be associated with the following:

- Ventricular tachyarrhythmia (ventricular fibrillation [VF] or a sustained type of ventricular tachycardia [VT])
- Ventricular standstill (brady-asystolic patterns)
- Electromechanical dissociation (EMD)

The term *pulseless electrical activity,* adopted by the Advanced Cardiac Life Support (ACLS) committee, refers to brady-asystolic patterns or EMD. The ECG patterns seen in cardiac arrest are briefly reviewed in the following sections, with emphasis placed on their clinical implications (Figs. 17.1 to 17.6).

VENTRICULAR TACHYARRHYTHMIA

With VF the ventricles do not contract but instead twitch rapidly in a completely ineffective way. No cardiac output occurs, and the patient loses consciousness within seconds. The characteristic ECG pattern, with its unmistakable fast oscillatory waves, is illustrated in Fig. 17.1.

Of the three basic ECG patterns seen with cardiac arrest, VF is the most common one initially encountered. It may appear spontaneously, although as noted in Chapter 14, it often is preceded by another ventricular arrhythmia (usually VT or premature ventricular beats). Fig. 17.2 shows a VT degenerating into VF during cardiac arrest.

The treatment of VF was mentioned in Chapter 12. The patient should be immediately defibrillated, with a *defibrillator (cardioverter)* used to administer a direct-current electric shock to the heart by means of paddles placed on the chest wall (see Chapter 14). An example of successful defibrillation is presented in Fig. 17.6, *D.*

Success in defibrillating any patient depends on a number of factors. The single most important factor is haste: the less delay in defibrillation, the greater the chance of succeeding.

Sometimes repeated shocks must be administered before the patient is successfully defibrillated. In other cases all attempts fail. Finally, external cardiac compression *must* be continued between attempts at defibrillation.

Cardiac arrest may also occur during a sustained episode of other ventricular tachyarrhythmias, including conventional VT, torsade de pointes, and ventricular flutter (see Chapter 14).*

VENTRICULAR STANDSTILL (BRADY-ASYSTOLIC PATTERNS)

Ventricular standstill and escape rhythms are described in Chapter 11. The normal pacemaker of the heart is the sinus node, which is located in the right atrium. Failure of the sinus node to function (sinus arrest) leads to ventricular standstill (asystole) if no other subsidiary pacemaker (e.g., in the atria, AV junction, or ventricles) takes over. In such cases the ECG records a *straight-line pattern* (see Fig. 17.3), indicating asystole. Whenever you encounter a straight-line pattern, you need to confirm this finding in at least two leads and check to see that all electrodes are connected to the patient. Electrodes often become disconnected during a cardiac arrest, leading to the mistaken diagnosis of asystole. Very low-amplitude VF may also mimic a straight-line pattern.

The treatment of ventricular standstill also requires continued external cardiac compression. Sometimes spontaneous cardiac electrical activity resumes. Drugs such as epinephrine may help stimulate cardiac activity. Patients with refractory ventricular standstill require a *temporary pacemaker,* which may be inserted at the bedside in an emergency situation. As described in Chapter 20, the temporary *transvenous* pacemaker is a special catheter wire electrode that is usually inserted

---

*Sometimes a strong thump on the sternum with your fist ("thump version") may restore normal rhythm during cardiac arrest, particularly if the patient is having a sustained run of VT or VF and a defibrillator is not immediately available.

Fig. 17.1 Ventricular fibrillation causing cardiac arrest.

VT   VF

Fig. 17.2 Ventricular tachycardia *(VT)* and ventricular fibrillation *(VF)* recorded during cardiac arrest. The rapid sine-wave type of ventricular tachycardia seen here is sometimes referred to as *ventricular flutter.*

Fig. 17.3 Complete ventricular standstill (asystole) producing a straight-line pattern during cardiac arrest.

Cardiac Arrest: Brady-Asystolic Patterns

A

B

Fig. 17.4 Escape rhythms with underlying ventricular standstill. **A,** Junctional escape rhythm with narrow QRS complexes. **B,** Idioventricular escape rhythm with wide QRS complexes. Treatment should include the use of intravenous atropine and, if needed, sympathomimetic drugs in an attempt to speed up these bradycardias, which cannot support the circulation. If hyperkalemia is present, it should be vigorously treated.

Fig. 17.5 External cardiac compression artifact. External cardiac compression during a resuscitation produces artifactual ECG complexes *(C)*, which may be mistaken for *QRS* complexes.

Fig. 17.6 ECG history of cardiac arrest and successful resuscitation. The left panel shows the ECG sequence during an actual cardiac arrest. The right panel shows sequential therapy appropriate for the different ECG patterns. **A** and **B,** Initially the ECG showed ventricular standstill (asystole) with a straight-line pattern, which was treated by external cardiac compression. **C** and **D,** Next ventricular fibrillation was seen. **E** to **G,** Sinus rhythm appeared after defibrillation with 400 watt-seconds of direct-current electric shock. (*C,* external cardiac compression artifact; *R,* R wave from the spontaneous QRS complex; *DC,* direct current; *V,* ventricular premature beat.)

through a vein into the right ventricle and connected to a battery outside the body. A type of *external* temporary pacemaker that does not require intravenous insertion is also commercially available. This noninvasive *(transcutaneous)* pacemaker uses special electrodes that are pasted on the chest wall. However, transcutaneous pacing may not always be effective, and it may be quite painful in conscious patients.

Not uncommonly with ventricular standstill, you also see occasional QRS complexes appearing at infrequent intervals against the background of the basic straight-line rhythm. These are *escape beats* and represent the attempt of intrinsic cardiac pacemakers to restart the heart's beat (see Chapter 11). Examples of escape rhythms with underlying ventricular standstill are shown in Fig. 17.4. In some cases the escape beats are narrow, indicating their origin from either the atria or the AV junction (Fig. 17.4, *A*). In others they come from a lower focus in the ventricles, producing a slow *idioventricular* rhythm with wide QRS complexes (see Fig. 17.4, *B*). The term *brady-asystolic pattern* is used to describe this type of cardiac arrest ECG.

Escape beats should not be confused with *artifacts* produced by external cardiac compression. Artifacts are large, wide deflections that occur with each compression (see Fig. 17.5). Their size varies with the strength of the compression, and their direction varies with the lead in which they appear (i.e., usually negative in leads II, III, and aV_F, positive in leads aV_R and aV_L).

ELECTROMECHANICAL DISSOCIATION

In the large majority of patients with cardiac arrest the ECG shows either a sustained ventricular tachyarrhythmia (VF or VT) or a brady-asystolic pattern. Occasionally, however, the ECG of patients in cardiac arrest surprisingly continues to show identifiable, narrow QRS complexes at a relatively physiologic rate. The actual heart rhythm in such cases may be a sinus rhythm, AV junctional (nodal) rhythm, AF, or other supraventricular mechanism. However, despite the presence of recurring QRS complexes and even P waves on the ECG, the patient is unconscious and does not have a palpable pulse or blood pressure detectable by usual clinical methods. In other words, the patient has cardiac electrical activity but insufficient mechanical heart contractions to pump blood effectively. The term *electromechanical dissociation (EMD)* is used in such cases.

EMD can arise in a number of settings. When assessing a patient with EMD, you must consider potentially *reversible* causes first. These include *severe hypovolemia, hypoxemia,* and *acidosis.* Another important reversible cause of EMD is *pericardial (cardiac) tamponade,* in which pericardial effusion decreases cardiac output and ultimately causes cardiac arrest. Pericardial tamponade can be treated by removing some of the fluid from the pericardial sac with a special needle inserted through the chest wall *(pericardiocentesis).* Because the disease process is primarily extracardiac (i.e., involving the pericardium), the ECG generally shows relatively normal electrical activity, despite the impaired mechanical function of the heart. Low voltage with sinus tachycardia is often present. Electrical alternans may be seen (see Chapter 10). *Tension pneumothorax* and *massive pulmonary embolism* are two other potentially reversible causes of EMD.

One of the most common settings in which EMD occurs is when the myocardium has sustained severe generalized injury that may not be reversible, such as with myocardial infarction (MI). In such cases, even though the heart's conduction system may be intact enough to generate a relatively normal rhythm, the amount of functional ventricular muscle is insufficient to respond to this electrical signal with an adequate contraction. Sometimes the myocardial depression is temporary and reversible ("stunned myocardium"), and the patient may respond to resuscitative efforts.

In summary, the three basic ECG patterns seen with cardiac arrest are ventricular tachyarrhythmia, ventricular standstill (brady-asystolic patterns), and EMD. During the course of resuscitating any patient, you may see two or even all three of these ECG patterns at different times during the arrest. Fig. 17.6 shows the "ECG history" of a cardiac arrest.

Clinical Causes of Cardiac Arrest

Cardiac arrest associated with any of the three electrical mechanisms—ventricular tachyarrhythmia, ventricular standstill, or EMD—may occur in numerous settings. It can be due to any type of organic heart disease. For example, a patient with an acute MI may have cardiac arrest for several reasons. Myocardial ischemia and increased ventricular electrical instability may precipitate VF. Damage to the conduction system may result in ventricular standstill. Finally, EMD may occur with extensive myocardial injury. Occasionally, actual rupture of the infarcted ventricular wall occurs, leading to fatal pericardial tamponade. Cardiac arrest also occurs when electrical instability is associated with *chronic* heart disease resulting from previous infarction, valvular abnormalities, hypertension, or cardiomyopathy.

A lightning strike or an electric shock may produce cardiac arrest in the normal heart. Cardiac arrest may also occur during surgical procedures, particularly in patients with underlying heart disease. Drugs such as epinephrine can produce VF. Quinidine and related drugs may lead to torsade de pointes (see Chapter 14). Excessive digitalis can also lead to fatal ventricular arrhythmias (see Chapter 16). Hypokalemia and hypomagnesemia may potentiate arrhythmias associated with quinidine (and related drugs) or digitalis. Other cardiac drugs may precipitate sustained ventricular tachyarrhythmias through their so-called *pro-arrhythmic effect* (see Chapter 14). The recreational use of *cocaine* has also been reported to precipitate fatal arrhythmias.

Brady-asystolic cardiac arrest may occur with intrinsic conduction disease resulting from sick sinus syndrome (see Chapters 11 and 18) or with high-degree AV block (see Chapter 15). You need to exclude very important reversible causes of brady-asystolic arrest such as hyperkalemia (see Chapter 10) and drug toxicity (e.g., digitalis, tricyclic overdose, beta blockers, calcium channel blockers). Hypothermia may be associated with severe bradycardia. Conditions that may directly cause or contribute to pulseless electrical activity (brady-asystolic patterns or actual EMD) are summarized in Table 17.1.

Table 17.1 Conditions That Cause Pulseless Electrical Activity

Condition	Clues
Hypovolemia	History of blood or fluid loss, flat neck veins
Hypoxia	Cyanosis, abnormal blood gases, airway problems
Cardiac (pericardial) tamponade	History of trauma, renal failure or thoracic malignancy; no pulse with cardiopulmonary resuscitation, neck vein distension, impending tamponade (tachycardia, hypotension, low pulse pressure) changing to sudden bradycardia as the terminal event
Tension pneumothorax	History of asthma, ventilator use, chronic obstructive pulmonary disease, or trauma; no pulse with cardiopulmonary resuscitation, absent breath sounds, neck vein distension, tracheal deviation
Hypothermia	History of exposure to cold; low central body temperature
Massive pulmonary embolism	History, no pulse felt with cardiopulmonary resuscitation, distended neck veins
Drug overdose (tricyclic antidepressants, digoxin, beta blockers, calcium channel blockers)	Bradycardia, history of drug ingestion, empty medication bottles at the scene, neurologic examination
Hyperkalemia	ECG showing wide QRS complexes without P waves and then asystole; history of renal failure, diabetes, dialysis, or selected medications
Severe acidosis	History of preexisting acidosis, renal failure, diabetes mellitus
Acute, massive myocardial infarction	History, ECG, cardiac enzymes

From *Textbook of advanced cardiac life support*, Dallas, 1997, American Heart Association.

During and after successful resuscitation of the patient in cardiac arrest, an intensive search for the cause must be started. Serial 12-lead ECGs and serum cardiac enzyme levels are helpful in diagnosing MI. A complete blood count, serum electrolyte concentrations, and arterial blood gas measurements should be obtained. A portable chest x-ray unit and, if needed, an echocardiograph machine can be brought to the bedside. In addition, a pertinent medical history should be obtained from every available source, with particular attention to drug use (e.g., digitalis, antiarrhythmics, psychotropics, "recreational" drugs, etc.) and previous cardiac problems.

Sudden Cardiac Death

The term *sudden cardiac death* is used to describe the situation in which an individual who sustains a cardiac arrest and is not resuscitated dies instantly or within an hour or so of the development of symptoms. Over 400,000 such deaths occur each year in the United States. Sudden cardiac death is most often initiated by a ventricular tachyarrhythmia, less commonly by a brady-asystolic mechanism or EMD.

Most individuals with cardiac arrest have underlying structural heart disease. An estimated 20% of patients with acute MI die suddenly before reaching the hospital. Another important substrate for sudden death is severe left ventricular scarring from previous (chronic) MI or dilated cardiomyopathy. Other patients with sudden cardiac death have structural heart disease with valvular abnormalities or myocardial disease associated, for example, with aortic stenosis, hypertrophic cardiomyopathy, myocarditis, or right ventricular dysplasia.

Some patients with sudden cardiac death do not have mechanical cardiac dysfunction, but they may have intrinsic electrical instability as a result of long QT syndrome (predisposing to torsade de pointes), Wolff-Parkinson-White preexcitation syndrome, or conduction system disease causing heart block. As noted, drugs such as cocaine or cardiac antiarrhythmic agents may induce arrhythmias. Finally, a small subset of individuals sustain cardiac arrest without having any demonstrable structural or electrophysiologic abnormality.

The identification and management of patients at high risk for sudden death are central areas of investigation in cardiology today. The important role of *implantable cardioverter-defibrillator* devices in preventing sudden death in high-risk patients is mentioned in Chapter 14.

Review

Cardiac arrest occurs when the heart stops pumping blood. The diagnosis should be made clinically even before the patient is connected to an electrocardiograph. The major clinical sign of cardiac arrest is the absence of pulses in an unconscious patient.

Cardiac arrest may be associated with one or more of the following ECG patterns:

1. *Ventricular tachyarrhythmias* such as ventricular fibrillation, sustained typical ventricular tachycardia, torsade de pointes, or ventricular flutter
2. *Ventricular standstill (asystole)* or *brady-asystolic pattern,* which is a straight-line pattern, sometimes with interruptions by junctional or ventricular escape beats
3. *Electromechanical dissociation (EMD),* in which recurring QRS complexes and sometimes even P waves are not associated with a palpable pulse or blood pressure. EMD is usually caused by diffuse myocardial injury, although it may be due to pericardial tamponade, tension pneumothorax, or massive pulmonary embolism

Any or all of these patterns may be seen during the resuscitation of a patient in cardiac arrest.

With cardiac arrest the ECG may show distinctive *artifacts* caused by external cardiac compression. These large, wide deflections should not be mistaken for the intrinsic electrical activity of the heart.

The term *sudden cardiac death* is used in reference to individuals who sustain a cardiac arrest and, unless resuscitated, die instantly or within an hour or so of the development of symptoms.

Questions

1. Would a pacemaker be of any value in treating a patient with cardiac arrest and electromechanical dissociation?
2. The rhythm strip shown below was obtained from a patient during the course of a cardiac arrest and attempted resuscitation.
   a. What is the basic rhythm?
   b. What is the cause of the complexes marked *X*?

Monitor lead

3. Name four drugs that can produce cardiac arrest associated with a sustained ventricular tachyarrhythmia (i.e., ventricular fibrillation, monomorphic ventricular tachycardia, torsade de pointes, or ventricular flutter).

Bradycardias and Tachycardias
Review and differential diagnosis

*T*he preceding chapters described the major arrhythmias and atrioventricular (AV) conduction disturbances. These abnormalities can be classified in numerous ways. However, this chapter simply divides them into two groups—bradycardias and tachycardias—and discusses the differential diagnosis of each group.

Bradycardias (Bradyarrhythmias)

Several arrhythmias and conduction disturbances associated with a slow heart rate have been described. The term *bradycardia* (or *bradyarrhythmia*) refers to arrhythmias and conduction abnormalities that produce a heart rate of less than 60 beats/min. Fortunately, the differential diagnosis of a slow pulse is relatively simple in that only a few causes must be considered. Bradyarrhythmias fall into five general classes (box).

SINUS BRADYCARDIA
Sinus bradycardia is sinus rhythm with a rate less than 60 beats/min (Fig. 18.1).* Each QRS complex is preceded by a P wave; the P wave is negative in lead aV_R and positive in lead II, indicating that the sinoatrial (SA) node is the pacemaker. Some patients may have a sinus bradycardia of 40 beats/min or less.

Sinus bradycardia may be related to a decreased firing rate of the sinus node pacemaker cells or to actual SA block.* The most extreme example is SA node arrest (see Chapter 11).

AV JUNCTIONAL (NODAL) ESCAPE RHYTHM
With a slow AV junctional escape rhythm (Fig. 18.2) either the P waves (seen just before or just after the QRS complexes) are *retrograde* (inverted in lead II and upright in lead aV_R), or no P waves are apparent if the atria and ventricles are stimulated simultaneously.

AV HEART BLOCK (SECOND OR THIRD DEGREE) OR AV DISSOCIATION
A slow ventricular rate of 60 beats/min or less (even as low as 20 beats/min) is the rule with complete heart block because of the slow intrinsic rate of the junctional or idioventricular pacemaker (Fig. 18.3). In addition, patients with second-degree AV block (either Mobitz type I [Wenckebach] or Mobitz type II) often have a bradycardia because of the dropped beats (see Fig. 15.3 and Table 15.1). Isorhythmic AV dissociation, which may be confused with complete heart block, is also frequently associated with a heart rate of less than 60 beats/min (see Chapter 15).

---

*Some cardiologists reserve the term *sinus bradycardia* for rates less than 50 beats/min.

SA block refers to situations in which impulses formed in the sinus node fail to depolarize the atria.

Sinus Bradycardia

Fig. 18.1 Sinus bradycardia with a slight sinus arrhythmia.

AV Junctional Escape Rhythm

Fig. 18.2 The heart rate is about 43 beats/min. The baseline between the QRS complexes is perfectly flat (i.e., no P waves are evident).

Bradycardias: Simplified Classification

Sinus bradycardia, including sinoatrial block
Atrioventricular (AV) junctional (nodal) escape rhythm
AV heart block (second or third degree) or AV dissociation
Atrial fibrillation or flutter with a slow ventricular response
Idioventricular escape rhythm

ATRIAL FIBRILLATION OR FLUTTER WITH A SLOW VENTRICULAR RATE

Paroxysmal atrial fibrillation (AF) is generally associated with a rapid ventricular rate. However, the rate may become excessively slow (less than 50 to 60 beats/min) because of drug effects or toxicity (beta blockers, calcium channel blockers, digitalis) or because of underlying disease of the AV junction (Fig. 18.4). In such cases the ECG shows the characteristic atrial fibrillatory (f) waves with a slow ventricular (QRS) rate. The f waves may be very fine and easily overlooked. (A very slow, regularized ventricular response in AF suggests the presence of complete AV heart block; see Chapter 15.)

IDIOVENTRICULAR ESCAPE RHYTHM

When the SA nodal and AV junctional escape pacemakers fail to function, a very slow pacemaker in the ventricular conduction (His-Purkinje) system may take over. This rhythm is referred to as an *idioventricular escape rhythm.* The rate is usually very slow (less than 45 beats/min), and the QRS

Complete Heart Block

Fig. 18.3 The atrial (P wave) rate is about 80 beats/min. The ventricular (QRS) rate is about 43 beats/min. Because the atria and ventricles are beating independently, the PR intervals are variable. The QRS complex is wide because the ventricles are being paced by an idioventricular pacemaker.

Atrial Fibrillation with a Slow, Regularized Ventricular Rate

Fig. 18.4 Regularization and excessive slowing of the ventricular rate with atrial fibrillation are usually a sign of digitalis toxicity or intrinsic atrioventricular nodal disease (see Chapter 16).

complexes are wide without any preceding P wave (see Fig. 17.4, *B*). *In such cases, hyperkalemia should always be excluded.*

CLINICAL SIGNIFICANCE

With the exception of sinus bradycardia, which is a common normal variant, the other bradycardias are often abnormal.* The possible causes of AV junctional rhythms, heart block, and AF were described in earlier chapters.

Digitalis excess or other drug toxicity (e.g., beta blockers, calcium channel blockers) must always be considered in any patient with a bradycardia. Hyperkalemia is another important, reversible, life-threatening cause of bradyarrhythmias (see Chapter 10).

Patients with any of the bradycardias just discussed may have no symptoms, or they may complain of light-headedness or fainting because of decreased cardiac output. The treatment depends on the particular arrhythmia and the clinical setting.

In summary, most patients with an ECG heart rate of less than 60 beats/min have one of the five following classes of arrhythmia: sinus bradycardia (including SA block), AV junctional escape rhythm, AV heart block (or AV dissociation), AF or atrial flutter with a very slow ventricular rate, or idioventricular escape rhythm.*

Tachycardias (Tachyarrhythmias)

At the opposite end of the spectrum from bradyarrhythmias are the tachycardias. These rhythm disturbances produce a heart rate faster than

---

*Normal persons (in particular, athletes with increased vagal tone at rest) occasionally show a slow junctional rhythm or even Wenckebach AV block.

*Bradycardia can also be due to a wandering atrial pacemaker (see Fig. 18.15) or isorhythmic AV dissociation (see Fig. 15.8).

100 beats/min. The tachyarrhythmias can be usefully divided into two general groups: those with a "narrow" (normal) QRS duration and those with a "wide" QRS duration. Narrow-complex tachycardias are almost invariably *supra*ventricular (i.e., the focus of stimulation is within or *above* the AV junction). Wide-complex tachycardias, by contrast, are either ventricular or supraventricular with aberrant ventricular conduction (supraventricular tachycardia [SVT] with aberrancy).

The four major classes of supraventricular tachyarrhythmia* are sinus tachycardia, paroxysmal supraventricular tachycardia (PSVT), atrial flutter, and AF. With each class, cardiac activation occurs at one or more sites in the atria or AV junction (node), above the ventricles (hence *supra*ventricular). This is in contrast to ventricular tachycardia (VT), in which the stimulus starts in the ventricles themselves. VT is simply a run of three or more consecutive premature ventricular depolarizations (see Fig. 14.5). The QRS complexes are always wide because the ventricles are not being stimulated simultaneously. The rate of VT is usually between 100 and 200 beats/min. By contrast, with supraventricular arrhythmias the ventricles are stimulated normally (simultaneously), and the QRS complexes are therefore narrow (unless a bundle branch block is also present).

The first step in analyzing a tachyarrhythmia is to look at the width of the QRS complex in all 12 leads if possible. If the QRS complex is narrow (0.1 second or less), you are dealing with some type of supraventricular arrhythmia and not VT. If the QRS complex is very wide (particularly if greater than 0.14 second), you should consider the rhythm to be VT unless it can be proved otherwise.

---

*Be aware of possible confusion in terminology. Cardiologists use the term *supraventricular tachycardia (SVT)* in two related, but different ways. First, SVT refers most generally to any arrhythmia originating in area of the AV junction, atria, or SA node, above the ventricular conduction system (hence *supra*ventricular). Second, SVT is also used more specifically to refer to a class of often paroxysmal supraventricular tachycardias (PSVTs) originating in the region of the atria or AV junction (node). These PSVTs, caused by reentry or automaticity, are distinct from sinus tachycardia, AF, or atrial flutter (see Chapter 12).

DIFFERENTIAL DIAGNOSIS OF NARROW-COMPLEX TACHYARRHYTHMIAS

The characteristics of sinus tachycardia, PSVTs, AF, and atrial flutter have been described in previous chapters. *Sinus tachycardia* in adults generally produces a heart rate between 100 and 180 beats/min, with the higher rates (150 to 180 beats/min) generally occurring in association with exercise. If you find a narrow-complex tachycardia with a rate of 150 beats/min or more in a resting adult, you are most likely dealing with one of the other three types of (nonsinus) arrhythmias mentioned previously.

PSVT and *AF* can generally be distinguished on the basis of their regularity. PSVT resulting from AV nodal reentry or a concealed bypass tract is usually an almost perfectly regular tachycardia with a ventricular rate between 140 and 250 beats/min (see Chapter 12). AF, on the other hand, is distinguished by its irregularity. Remember that with rapid AF (Fig. 18.5) the f waves may not be clearly visible, but the diagnosis can be made in almost every case by noting the absence of P waves and the haphazardly irregular QRS complexes.

Atrial flutter is characterized by "sawtooth" flutter (F) waves between QRS complexes (Fig. 18.6). However, when atrial flutter is present with 2:1 block (e.g., the atrial rate is 300 beats/min and the ventricular response is 150 beats/min), the F waves are often hidden. Therefore atrial flutter at 150 beats/min can be confused with sinus tachycardia, PSVT, or AF (Fig. 18.7). AF can be excluded because atrial flutter with 2:1 conduction is generally very regular.

Nevertheless, the differential diagnosis of sinus tachycardia, PSVT with a ventricular rate of about 150 beats/min, AF, and atrial flutter can be a problem (see Fig. 18.7). One measure often used to help separate these arrhythmias is *carotid sinus massage (CSM).** Pressure on the carotid sinus produces a reflex increase in vagal tone. The effects of CSM on sinus tachycardia, reentrant-types of PSVT, and atrial flutter are described next.

---

*CSM is not without risks, particularly in elderly patients. Consult texts cited in the Bibliography for details on this maneuver and the use of adenosine in the differential diagnosis of tachycardias.

Atrial Fibrillation with a Rapid Ventricular Rate

Fig. 18.5 The ventricular rate is about 130 beats/min (13 QRS cycles in 6 seconds). Notice the characteristic haphazardly irregular rhythm.

Fig. 18.6 Atrial flutter with 2:1 conduction.

Sinus Tachycardia

Sinus tachycardia generally slows slightly with CSM. However, no abrupt change in heart rate usually occurs. Slowing of sinus tachycardia may make the P waves more evident. Sinus tachycardia generally begins and ends gradually, not abruptly.

Paroxysmal Supraventricular Tachycardia

PSVT resulting from AV nodal reentry (AVNRT) or atrioventricular reentry (AVRT) involving a concealed bypass tract usually has an *all-or-none* response to CSM. In successful cases it breaks suddenly, and sinus rhythm resumes during the CSM (see Fig. 12.7). At other times CSM has no effect, and the tachycardia continues at the same rate. In cases of PSVT caused by atrial tachycardia (AT), CSM may have no effect or may increase the degree of block, resulting in a rapid sequence of nonconducted P waves.

Atrial Flutter

CSM often increases the degree of block in atrial flutter, converting flutter with a 2:1 response to 3:1 or 4:1 flutter with a ventricular rate of 100 or 75 beats/min. Slowing of the ventricular rate unmasks the characteristic F waves (see Fig. 13.2).

MULTIFOCAL ATRIAL TACHYCARDIA

Another variant of PSVT that has not yet been specifically discussed is *multifocal atrial tachycardia (MAT)*. An example is shown in Fig. 18.8. This tachyarrhythmia is characterized by multiple ectopic foci stimulating the atria. The diagnosis of MAT requires the presence of three or more (nonsinus) P waves with different shapes at a rate of 100 or more per minute. The PR intervals often vary. MAT is usually seen in patients with chronic lung disease. Because the ventricular rate

Fig. 18.7 Four "look-alike" narrow-complex tachyarrhythmias (lead II). **A,** Sinus tachycardia. **B,** Atrial fibrillation. **C,** Paroxysmal supraventricular tachycardia resulting from atrioventricular nodal reentrant tachycardia. **D,** Atrial flutter with 2:1 block. When the ventricular rate is about 150 beats/min, these four arrhythmias may be difficult if not impossible to tell apart on the standard ECG, particularly from a single lead. In the example of sinus tachycardia the P waves can barely be seen. Next, notice that the irregularity of the atrial fibrillation is very subtle. In the example of paroxysmal supraventricular tachycardia the rate is quite regular without evident P waves. In the strip illustrating atrial flutter the flutter waves cannot be seen clearly.

Multifocal Atrial Tachycardia

Fig. 18.8 Note the rapidly occurring P waves showing variable shapes, variable PR intervals, or both.

Fig. 18.9 A, Atrial fibrillation with a left bundle branch block pattern. **B,** Ventricular tachycardia. Based on the ECG appearance differentiating supraventricular tachycardia with bundle branch block from actual ventricular tachycardia may be difficult and sometimes impossible.

is irregular and rapid, this arrhythmia is most likely to be mistaken for AF. MAT is caused by multiple atrial pacemakers firing in an unpredictable fashion. This is in contrast to classic AT, which typically involves only a single ectopic pacemaker in the atrium (see Chapter 12).

DIFFERENTIAL DIAGNOSIS OF VENTRICULAR TACHYCARDIA

Tachycardias are divided into SVTs and VT. This section briefly describes the differential diagnosis of VT. A tachycardia with widened QRS complexes indicates two possible diagnoses. The first and more important is VT, a potentially life-threatening arrhythmia.* As noted, VT is a consecutive run of three or more ventricular premature beats at a rate generally between 100 and 200 or more beats/min. It is usually very regular. The second possible cause of a tachycardia with widened QRS

complexes is so-called *SVT with aberration.* The term *aberration* simply means that some abnormality in ventricular activation is present and causing widened QRS complexes.

DIFFERENTIATION OF SUPRAVENTRICULAR TACHYCARDIA WITH ABERRANCY AND VENTRICULAR TACHYCARDIA

Aberrancy with an SVT has only two major mechanisms: bundle branch block and the Wolff-Parkinson-White (WPW) preexcitation syndrome.

Supraventricular Tachycardia with Bundle Branch Block

If any of the SVTs just discussed occurs in association with a bundle branch block, the ECG shows a wide-complex tachycardia that may be mistaken for VT. For example, a patient with sinus tachycardia, AF, atrial flutter, or PSVT and concomitant right bundle branch block (RBBB) or left bundle branch block (LBBB) has a wide-complex tachycardia.

Fig. 18.9, *A*, shows AF with a rapid ventricular response occurring in conjunction with LBBB. Fig. 18.9, *B*, shows an example of VT. Because the

*Most cases of VT are associated with a very wide QRS complex. More rarely VT may occur with a QRS complex that is only mildly prolonged, particularly if the arrhythmia originates in the upper part of the ventricular septum or fascicles.

arrhythmias look so similar, it can be difficult to tell them apart. The major distinguishing feature is the irregularity of the AF as opposed to the regularity of the VT. However, VT sometimes may be irregular.

You need to remember that in some cases of SVT with aberration, the bundle branch block is seen only during the episodes of tachycardia. Such rate-related bundle branch blocks are said to be *tachycardia dependent.*

Supraventricular Tachycardia with Wolff-Parkinson-White Preexcitation Syndrome

The second mechanism responsible for a wide-complex tachycardia is SVT with the WPW syndrome (see Chapter 10). As noted, patients with WPW preexcitation have an accessory pathway connecting the atria and ventricles, thus bypassing the AV node. Such patients are especially prone to a reentrant type of PSVT with narrow (normal) QRS complexes. Sometimes, however, particularly if AF or atrial flutter develops, a wide-complex tachycardia may result from conduction down the bypass tract at very high rates. This kind of wide-complex tachycardia obviously mimics VT. An example of WPW with AF is shown in Fig. 18.10.

WPW with AF should be strongly suspected if you encounter a wide-complex tachycardia that is irregular and has a very high rate (very short RR intervals). In particular, RR intervals of 0.20 second or less are rarely seen with conventional AF or VT. These very short RR intervals are related to the ability of the bypass tract (in contrast to the AV node) to conduct impulses in extremely rapid succession (Fig. 18.10, *A*).

The recognition of WPW with AF is of considerable clinical importance because digitalis may paradoxically enhance conduction down the bypass tract. As a result the ventricular response may increase, leading to possible myocardial ischemia and in some cases to ventricular fibrillation. A similar effect has been reported with intravenous verapamil.

Diagnostic Clues

AV dissociation is an important clue that may be helpful in differentiating SVT with aberrancy

from VT. Recall from Chapter 15 that with AV dissociation the atria and ventricles are paced from separate sites. Some patients with VT also have AV dissociation; in other words, the ventricles are paced from an *ectopic* site at a rapid rate, while the atria continue to be paced independently by the SA node. In such cases you may be able to see P waves occurring at a slower rate than the rapid wide QRS complexes as shown in Fig. 18.11. Some of the P waves may be buried in the QRS complexes and therefore difficult to discern.

Unfortunately, only a minority of patients with VT clearly show AV dissociation. Therefore the absence of AV dissociation does not exclude VT. However, the presence of AV dissociation in a patient with wide QRS complexes at a rapid rate is virtually diagnostic of VT. Furthermore, in some cases of VT with AV dissociation the SA node may transiently "capture" the ventricles, producing a *capture beat,* which has a normal QRS duration, or a *fusion beat,* in which the sinus and ventricular beats coincide to produce a hybrid complex. Fig. 18.12 illustrates capture and fusion beats occurring with VT.

What other ECG clues are helpful in distinguishing SVT with aberration from VT? Over the years cardiologists have tried to develop more precise criteria to assist in this important differential diagnosis. Unfortunately, no single criterion has proved absolutely reliable. Nevertheless, in addition to AV dissociation, two other ECG clues can be helpful if you are confronted with a wide-complex tachycardia:

1. When the QRS shape resembles an RBBB pattern, an rsR′ in lead V_1 suggests SVT and a single broad R wave or a qR, QR, or RS complex in that lead suggests VT (Fig. 18.13).
2. When the QRS shape resembles an LBBB pattern, a prominent R wave in lead V_1 or V_2 or a QR complex in lead V_6 strongly suggests VT.

At times you may find it impossible to distinguish reliably between VT and SVT with aberration from the 12-lead ECG. In such cases clinical judgment must be used. For example, if the patient is hypotensive, the tachycardia is generally treated as VT (Table 18.1). On the other hand, remember that not all patients with VT are hypotensive. Indeed,

Fig. 18.10 A, Atrial fibrillation with the Wolff-Parkinson-White preexcitation syndrome may lead to a wide-complex tachycardia that has a very rapid rate. Notice that some of the RR intervals are less than 0.20 second. Irregularity is due to the underlying atrial fibrillation. **B,** After the arrhythmia has been converted to sinus rhythm, the classic triad of the Wolff-Parkinson-White syndrome is visible but subtle: relatively short PR interval, wide QRS complex, and delta wave (*arrow* in lead V$_3$).

Ventricular Tachycardia: AV Dissociation

Fig. 18.11 Sustained monomorphic ventricular tachycardia with atrioventricular (AV) dissociation. Note the independence of the atrial (sinus) rate (75 per minute) and ventricular (QRS) rate (140 per minute). The visible sinus P waves are indicated by ●, and the hidden P waves are indicated by ○.

Ventricular Tachycardia: Fusion and Capture Beats

Fig. 18.12 Sustained monomorphic ventricular tachycardia with atrioventricular dissociation producing fusion *(F)* and capture *(C)* beats. Leads I and II were recorded simultaneously.

Narrow QRS complexes	**Wide QRS complexes**

Sinus tachycardia
Paroxysmal supraven-
   tricular tachycardias*
Atrial flutter
Atrial fibrillation
	Ventricular tachycardia
	Supraventricular tachycardia
	   with aberration caused by
	   a bundle branch block or
	   Wolff-Parkinson-White
	   preexcitation syndrome

Table 18.1 **Major Tachyarrhythmias: Simplified Classification**

*The three most common types of paroxysmal supraventricular tachycardias are atrioventricular nodal reentrant tachycardias (AVNRTs), bypass-tract tachycardias, and atrial tachycardias (including paroxysmal atrial tachycardia and multifocal atrial tachycardia), as discussed in Chapter 12. Other *non*paroxysmal supraventricular tachycardias may also occur, including types of so-called *incessant* atrial, junctional, and bypass-tract tachycardias. (For further details, see texts cited in the Bibliography.)

occasional patients may have minimal symptoms at rest when they are in sustained VT.

You must remember that *intravenously administered verapamil should not be used in undiagnosed wide-complex tachycardias.* This drug may cause hemodynamic collapse in patients with VT or AF with WPW preexcitation syndrome.

Clinical Significance

As mentioned previously, the first question to ask in looking at any tachyarrhythmia is whether the rhythm is VT. If sustained VT is present, emergency treatment is required (see Chapter 14).

The treatment of narrow-complex tachycardias depends on the clinical setting. In patients with sinus tachycardia (see Chapter 11), treatment is directed at the underlying cause (e.g., fever, sepsis, congestive heart failure, or hyperthyroidism). Similarly, the treatment of MAT should be directed at the underlying problem (usually chronic pulmonary disease). Direct-current electrical cardioversion should *not* be used with MAT because it is unlikely to be helpful and it may induce serious ventricular arrhythmias. A calcium channel blocker (verapamil or diltiazem) can be used to slow the ventricular response in MAT.

In assessing any patient with a narrow-complex tachycardia, you should ask the following three key questions about the effects of the tachycardia on the heart and circulation:

1. Is the patient's blood pressure abnormally low? In particular, is the patient in shock?
2. Is the patient having an acute myocardial infarction or severe ischemia?
3. Is the patient in severe congestive heart failure (pulmonary edema)?

Patients in any one of these categories who have AF or atrial flutter with a rapid ventricular response or a PSVT require emergency therapy. If they do not respond promptly to initial drug therapy, electrical cardioversion should be considered.

Another major question to ask about any patient with a tachyarrhythmia (or any arrhythmia for that matter) is whether digitalis

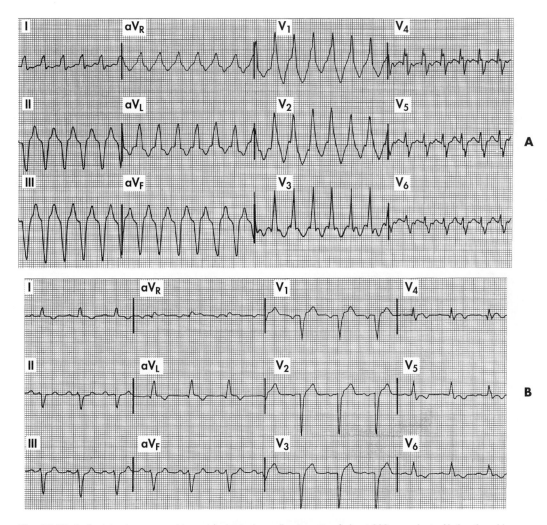

Fig. 18.13 A, Sustained monomorphic ventricular tachycardia at a rate of about 200 per minute. Notice the wide QRS complexes with a right bundle branch block morphology. The QRS complex in leads V$_1$ and V$_2$ shows a broad R wave. **B,** Following conversion to sinus rhythm, the pattern of an underlying anterior wall myocardial infarction and ventricular aneurysm becomes evident. Q waves and ST elevations are seen in leads in V$_1$, V$_2$, and V$_3$; ischemic T wave inversions are present in leads V$_4$, V$_5$, and V$_6$. Note also that the QRS complex is wide (0.12 second) because of an intraventricular conduction delay with left axis deviation (left anterior hemiblock). The prominent negative P waves in lead V$_1$ are due to left atrial abnormality.

or other drugs are part of the therapeutic regimen. Some arrhythmias (e.g., AT with block) may be digitalis-toxic rhythms, disturbances for which electrical cardioversion is contraindicated (see Chapter 16).

Sick Sinus Syndrome and the Brady-Tachy Syndrome

An interesting group of patients has bradyarrhythmia sometimes alternating with episodes of tachyarrhythmia. The term *sick sinus syndrome* was coined to describe patients with SA node dysfunction that causes marked sinus bradycardia or sinus arrest, sometimes with junctional escape rhythms, which may lead to symptoms of lightheadedness and even syncope.

In some patients with sick sinus syndrome, bradycardia episodes are interspersed with paroxysms of tachycardia (usually AF, atrial flutter, or some type of PSVT). Sometimes the bradycardia occurs immediately after spontaneous termination of the tachycardia. The term *brady-tachy syndrome* has been used to describe patients with sick

sinus syndrome who have both tachyarrhythmias and bradyarrhythmias (Fig. 18.14).

The diagnosis of sick sinus syndrome and, in particular, the brady-tachy variant often requires monitoring the patient's heartbeat over several hours or even days. A single ECG strip may be normal or may reveal only the bradycardic or tachycardic episode. Treatment generally requires a permanent pacemaker to prevent sinus arrest and antiarrhythmic drugs to control the tachycardias after the pacemaker has been inserted.

Brady-Tachy Syndrome

Fig. 18.14 Brady-tachy (sick sinus) syndrome. This rhythm strip shows a narrow-complex tachycardia (probably atrial flutter) followed by a prominent sinus pause, two sinus beats, an atrioventricular junctional escape beat *(J)*, and then sinus rhythm again.

Wandering Atrial Pacemaker

Lead II (continuous)

Fig. 18.15 The variability of the P wave configuration in this lead II rhythm strip is caused by shifting of the pacemaker site between the sinus node and ectopic atrial locations.

Wandering Atrial Pacemaker

Wandering atrial pacemaker is an arrhythmia that is somewhat difficult to classify. As shown in Fig. 18.15, this arrhythmia is characterized by multiple P waves of varying configuration with a relatively normal or slow heart rate. This pattern reflects shifting of the pacemaker between the SA node, other atrial sites, and sometimes the AV junction. Wandering atrial pacemaker may be seen in a variety of settings. Occasionally it develops in normal persons (particularly during sleep). It may also occur with digitalis excess or other drug toxicity, sick sinus syndrome, and different types of organic heart disease.

Wandering atrial pacemaker is distinct from MAT, another arrhythmia with multiple different P waves. In wandering atrial pacemaker the rate is normal or slow. In MAT it is rapid.

Review

Arrhythmias can be grouped into *bradycardias* (heart rate *slower* than 60 beats/min) and *tachycardias* (heart rate *faster* than 100 beats/min).

Bradycardias include five major classes of arrhythmias or conduction disturbances:

1. Sinus bradycardia
2. Atrioventricular (AV) junctional (nodal) escape rhythm
3. Second- or third-degree heart block or AV dissociation
4. Atrial fibrillation or flutter with a slow ventricular rate
5. Idioventricular escape rhythm.

Digitalis or other drug toxicity, or hyperkalemia, may be responsible for any of these arrhythmias.

Tachycardias can be subdivided into those with *narrow* QRS complexes and those with *wide* QRS complexes. The narrow-complex QRS tachycardias are almost always *supraventricular* in origin and include the following:

1. Sinus tachycardia
2. Paroxysmal supraventricular tachycardias (PSVTs), including atrial tachycardia (AT), AV nodal reentrant tachycardia (AVNRT), and AV reentrant tachycardia (AVRT) (see Chapter 12).
3. Atrial fibrillation
4. Atrial flutter

Carotid sinus massage is sometimes helpful in differentiating these arrhythmias at the bedside. Tachycardias with wide QRS complexes may be either *ventricular* or any of the supraventricular tachycardias associated with a *bundle branch block* or *Wolff-Parkinson-White* preexcitation mechanism.

The term *sick sinus syndrome* describes patients with sinoatrial node dysfunction who have a marked sinus bradycardia, sometimes with sinus arrest or slow junctional rhythms, that causes light-headedness or syncope. Some patients with sick sinus syndrome have periods of tachycardia alternating with the bradycardia *(brady-tachy syndrome).*

Wandering atrial pacemaker is an arrhythmia characterized by multiple P waves of varying configuration, usually with a relatively normal or slow heart rate.

Questions

1. Answer the following questions about the lead II rhythm strip below:
   a. Is the rate regular or irregular?
   b. Are discrete P waves present?
   c. What is this arrhythmia?

2. What is the most likely diagnosis for the arrhythmia shown in this monitor lead?

3. A 40-year-old woman complaining of occasional palpitations with a fast heartbeat is found to have runs of narrow QRS complex tachycardia at a rate of 200 beats/min without evident P waves on his Holter monitor tracing. The rhythm is very regular. What is the most likely diagnosis?
4. What is the cause of the bradycardia in the rhythm strip shown below?

5. Name three readily reversible causes of bradycardia.

Limitations and Uses of the ECG

*T*hroughout this book the clinical uses of the ECG have been stressed. This review chapter underscores some important *limitations* of the ECG, reemphasizes its *utility*, and reviews some common *pitfalls* in its interpretation.

Important Limitations of the ECG

Like most clinical tests the ECG yields both *false-positive* and *false-negative* results. A false-positive result is an apparently abnormal ECG in a normal subject. For example, prominent precordial voltage may occur in the absence of left ventricular hypertrophy (LVH) (see Chapter 6). Furthermore, Q waves may occur as a normal variant and therefore do not always indicate heart disease (see Chapter 8). False-negative results, on the other hand, occur when the ECG fails to show evidence of some cardiac abnormality. For example, some patients with acute myocardial infarction (MI) may not show diagnostic ST-T changes, and patients with severe coronary artery disease may not show diagnostic ST depressions during stress testing.

The diagnostic accuracy of any test is determined by the percentages of false-positive and false-negative results. The *sensitivity* of a test is a measure of the percentage of patients with a particular abnormality that can be identified by an abnormal test result. For example, a test with 100% sensitivity has no false-negative results. The more false-negative results, the less sensitive is the test. The *specificity* of a test is a measure of the percentage of false-positive results. The more false-positive test results, the less specific is the test.

As just noted, both the sensitivity and specificity of the ECG in diagnosing a variety of condi-

tions, including MI, are limited. Clinicians need to be aware of these diagnostic limitations. The following are some important problems that *cannot* be excluded simply because the ECG is normal or shows only nondiagnostic abnormalities:

- Prior MI
- Acute MI*
- Severe coronary artery disease
- Significant LVH
- Significant right ventricular hypertrophy (RVH)
- Intermittent arrhythmias such as paroxysmal atrial fibrillation (AF), paroxysmal supraventricular tachycardia (PSVT), ventricular tachycardia (VT), and bradycardias
- Acute pulmonary embolism
- Pericarditis

Utility of the ECG in Special Cases

Although the ECG has definite limitations, it often helps in the diagnosis of specific cardiac conditions and sometimes aids in the evaluation and management of general medical problems such as life-threatening electrolyte disorders (box). Some particular areas in which the ECG may be helpful are as follows:

- *Myocardial infarction*
  Most patients with acute MI show diagnostic ECG changes (i.e., new Q waves and/or ST elevations, hyperacute T waves, ST depressions, or T wave inversions). However, in the weeks and months after an acute MI these changes

---

*The pattern of acute MI may also be masked in patients with left bundle branch block, Wolff-Parkinson-White preexcitation syndrome, or electronic ventricular pacemakers.

may become less apparent and in some cases may disappear.

ST segment elevation in a right chest precordial lead (e.g., V_{4R}) in a patient with acute inferior infarction indicates associated right ventricular ischemia or infarction (see Chapter 8).

Persistent ST elevations several weeks after an MI should suggest a ventricular aneurysm.

- *Pulmonary embolism*

A new S_IQ_{III} or right bundle branch block pattern, particularly in association with sinus tachycardia, should suggest the possibility of acute cor pulmonale resulting from, for example, pulmonary embolism (see Chapter 10).

- *Pericardial tamponade*

Low QRS voltage in a patient with elevated central venous pressure (distended neck veins) and sinus tachycardia suggests possible pericardial tamponade. Sinus tachycardia with electrical alternans is virtually diagnostic of pericardial effusion with tamponade (see Chapter 10).

- *Aortic valve disease*

LVH is seen in most patients with critical aortic stenosis or severe aortic regurgitation.

- *Mitral valve disease*

ECG signs of left atrial enlargement (abnormality) and RVH strongly suggest mitral stenosis (Fig. 19.1).

Frequent ventricular premature beats (VPBs) and nonspecific ST-T changes, particularly in a younger patient, should prompt a search for mitral valve prolapse.

- *Atrial septal defect*

Most patients with a moderate to large atrial septal defect have a right bundle branch block pattern.

- *Hyperkalemia*

Severe hyperkalemia, a life-threatening electrolyte abnormality, virtually always produces ECG changes, beginning with T wave peaking, loss of P waves, QRS widening, and finally asystole (see Chapter 10).

- *Renal failure*

The triad of LVH (caused by hypertension), peaked T waves (caused by hyperkalemia), and prolonged QT interval (caused by hypocalcemia) should suggest chronic renal failure.

ECG as a Clue to Acute Life-Threatening Conditions without Primary Heart or Lung Disease

Cerebrovascular accident (especially intracranial bleed)
Drug toxicity
    Tricyclic antidepressant overdose
Electrolyte disorders
    Hypokalemia
    Hyperkalemia
    Hypocalcemia
    Hypercalcemia
Endocrine disorders
    Hypothyroidism
    Hyperthyroidism
Hypothermia

- *Thyroid disease*

The combination of low voltage and sinus bradycardia should suggest possible *hypothyroidism*. ("Low and slow—think hypo.")

Unexplained AF (or sinus tachycardia at rest) should prompt a search for *hyperthyroidism*.

- *Chronic lung disease*

The combination of low voltage and poor precordial R wave progression is commonly seen with chronic obstructive lung disease.

- *Cardiomyopathy*

The ECG-CHF (congestive heart failure) triad of relatively low limb lead voltage, prominent precordial voltage, and poor R wave progression suggests an underlying dilated cardiomyopathy (see Chapter 10).

Common Applications of the ECG

The ECG may also provide important clues in the evaluation of such major medical problems as syncope, coma, shock, and weakness.

SYNCOPE

Fainting can result from primary cardiac factors and various noncardiac causes. The primary cardiac causes can be divided into mechanical obstructions (aortic stenosis, primary pulmonary hypertension, or atrial myxoma) and electrical problems

Fig. 19.1 This ECG from a 45-year-old woman with severe mitral stenosis shows multiple abnormalities. The rhythm is sinus tachycardia. Right axis deviation and a tall R wave in lead V_1 indicate right ventricular hypertrophy. The prominent biphasic P wave in lead V_1 indicates left atrial enlargement. The tall P waves in lead II may indicate concomitant right atrial enlargement. Nonspecific ST-T changes and incomplete right bundle branch block are also present. The combination of right ventricular hypertrophy and left atrial enlargement is highly suggestive of mitral stenosis.

(bradyarrhythmias or tachyarrhythmias). The noncardiac causes of syncope include neurogenic mechanisms (e.g., vasovagal attacks), orthostatic (postural) hypotension, and brain dysfunction from vascular insufficiency or metabolic derangements (e.g., from alcohol or hypoglycemia).

Patients with syncope resulting from aortic stenosis generally show LVH on their resting ECG. Primary pulmonary hypertension is most common in young and middle-aged adult women. The ECG generally shows RVH. The presence of frequent VPBs may be a clue to intermittent VT. Evidence of previous Q wave MI should suggest the possibility of sustained monomorphic VT. Syncope with QT(U) prolongation should suggest *torsade de pointes,* a potentially lethal ventricular arrhythmia (see Chapter 14). A severe bradycardia (usually from heart block or sick sinus syndrome) in a patient with syncope constitutes the Stokes-Adams syndrome (see Chapter 15). In some cases, serious arrhythmias can be detected only when long-term monitoring is performed. Syncope in a patient with ECG evidence of bifascicular block (e.g., RBBB with left anterior hemiblock) should prompt a search for intermittent second- or third-degree heart block or other arrhythmias. Syncope in patients taking quinidine, sotalol, and related drugs may be associated with torsade de pointes or other arrhythmias.

Selected patients with *unexplained syncope* may benefit from invasive electrophysiologic testing. During these studies the placement of intracardiac electrodes permits more direct and controlled assessment of sinoatrial (SA) node function, atrioventricular (AV) conduction, and the susceptibility to sustained ventricular or supraventricular tachycardias.

COMA

An ECG should be obtained in all comatose patients. If coma is from MI with subsequent cardiac arrest, diagnostic ECG changes related to the infarct are usually seen. Subarachnoid hemorrhage may cause very deep T wave inversions (see Fig. 9.10), simulating the changes of MI. When coma is associated with hypercalcemia, the QT interval is often short. Myxedema coma generally presents with ECG evidence of sinus bradycardia and low voltage. Widening of the QRS complex in a comatose patient should always raise the possibility of drug overdose (tricyclic antidepressant or phenothiazine) or hyperkalemia.

SHOCK

An ECG should be obtained promptly in patients with severe hypotension because MI is a major cause of shock (cardiogenic shock). In other cases, hypotension may be caused or worsened by a bradyarrhythmia or tachyarrhythmia. Finally, some patients with shock from noncardiac causes (e.g., hypovolemia or diabetic ketoacidosis) may have myocardial ischemia and sometimes MI as a *consequence* of their initial problem.

WEAKNESS

An ECG may be helpful in evaluating patients with unexplained weakness. Elderly patients, in particular, may have relatively "silent" MIs with minimal or atypical symptoms, such as the onset of fatigue or general weakness. Distinctive ECG changes may also occur with certain pharmacologic and metabolic factors (e.g., hypokalemia or hypocalcemia) that cause weakness.

Common Pitfalls in ECG Interpretation

You can minimize errors in interpreting ECGs by taking care to analyze *all* the points listed in the first section of Chapter 21. Many mistakes result from the failure to be systematic. Other mistakes result from confusing ECG patterns that are "look-alikes." Important reminders are provided in the accompanying box. Some common pitfalls in ECG interpretation are discussed in the following sections.

Unless recognized and corrected, inadvertent reversal of limb lead electrodes can cause diagnostic confusion. For example, reversal of the left and right arm electrodes can cause an apparent right-

---

Some Important Reminders

Check standardization.

Exclude limb lead reversal. (For example, a negative P wave with a negative QRS complex in lead I suggests a left/right arm electrode switch.)

Look for hidden P waves, which may indicate atrioventricular (AV) block, blocked atrial premature beats, or atrial tachycardia with block.

With a regular narrow-complex tachycardia at about 150 beats/min at rest, consider atrial flutter with 2 : 1 block versus paroxysmal supraventricular tachycardia or (less likely) sinus tachycardia.

With group beating (clusters of QRS complexes), consider Mobitz type I (Wenckebach) block or blocked atrial premature beats.

With wide QRS complexes and with short PR intervals, consider the Wolff-Parkinson-White preexcitation pattern.

With wide QRS complexes without P waves or with AV block, think of hyperkalemia.

---

ward QRS axis shift as well as an abnormal P wave axis that simulates an ectopic atrial or junctional rhythm (Fig. 19.2). As a general rule, *when lead I shows a negative P wave and a negative QRS, reversal of the left and right arm electrodes should be suspected.*

Voltage can appear abnormal if standardization is not checked. Many ECGs are mistakenly thought to show "high" or "low" voltage when the voltage is actually normal but the standardization marker is set at half standardization or two-times normal sensitivity.

Atrial flutter with 2 : 1 block is one of the most commonly missed diagnoses. The rhythm is often misdiagnosed as sinus tachycardia (mistaking part of a flutter wave for a P wave) or PSVT. *When you see a narrow-complex tachycardia with a ventricular rate of about 150 beats/min, you should always consider atrial flutter* (see Fig. 13.2).

Coarse atrial fibrillation and atrial flutter are sometimes confused. When the fibrillatory (f) waves are prominent (coarse), the rhythm is commonly mistaken for atrial flutter. However, with AF the ventricular rate is completely erratic, and the atrial waves are not exactly consistent from one segment to the next. With pure atrial flutter the atrial waves are identical from one moment to

Lead Reversal

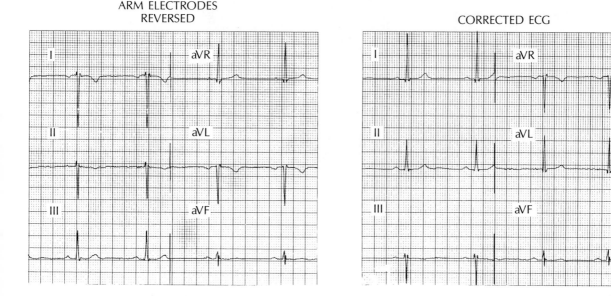

Fig. 19.2 Whenever the QRS axis is unusual, limb lead reversal may be the problem. Most commonly, the left and right arm electrodes become switched so that lead I shows a negative P wave and a negative QRS complex.

the next, even when the ventricular response is variable. (Fig 19.3).

The Wolff-Parkinson-White pattern is frequently mistaken for bundle branch block, hypertrophy, or infarction because the preexcitation results in a wide QRS complex and may cause increased QRS voltage, T wave inversions, and pseudoinfarction Q waves (see Fig. 10.20).

Isorhythmic AV dissociation and complete heart block can be confused. With isorhythmic AV dissociation the SA and AV node pacemakers become "desynchronized," and the QRS rate is the same as or slightly faster than the P wave rate (see Chapter 15). With complete heart block the atria and ventricles also beat independently, but the ventricular rate is much slower than the atrial (sinus) rate. Isorhythmic AV dissociation is usually a minor arrhythmia although it may reflect conduction disease or drug toxicity (e.g., digitalis, diltiazem, verapamil, and beta blockers). Complete heart block is always a major arrhythmia and generally requires pacemaker therapy.

Normal-variant and pathologic Q waves require special attention. Remember that Q waves may be a normal variant as part of QS waves in leads aV_R, aV_L, aV_F, III, V_1, and occasionally V_2 (see Chapter 8). Small q waves (as part of qR waves) may occur in leads I, II, III, aV_L, and aV_F as well as in the left chest leads (V_4 to V_6). These "septal" Q waves are less than 0.04 second in duration. On the other hand, small pathologic Q waves may be overlooked because they are not always very deep. In some cases it may not be possible to state definitively whether or not a Q wave is pathologic.

Mobitz type I (Wenckebach) AV block is a commonly missed diagnosis. "Group beating" is an important clue to the diagnosis of this problem (see Chapter 15). The QRS complexes become grouped in clusters because of the intermittent failure of AV nodal conduction.

Hidden P waves may lead to mistakes in the diagnosis of a number of arrhythmias, including blocked APBs, paroxysmal AT with block, and

Fig. 19.3 Atrial flutter with variable block **(A)** and coarse atrial fibrillation **(B)** are often confused. Notice that with atrial fibrillation the ventricular rate is completely erratic and the atrial waves are not identical from segment to segment.

second- or third-degree (complete) AV block. Therefore you must search the ST segment and T wave for buried P waves (see Fig. 16.3).

Multifocal atrial tachycardia (MAT) and AF are often confused because the ventricular response in both is usually rapid and irregular. With MAT, you need to look for multiple different P waves. With AF, you must be careful not to mistake the sometimes "coarse" f waves for actual P waves.

LBBB may be mistaken for infarction because it is associated with poor R wave progression and often ST segment elevation in the right chest leads.

U waves are sometimes overlooked. Small U waves are a physiologic finding, but large U waves (which may be apparent in only the chest leads) are sometimes an important marker of hypokalemia or drug toxicity (e.g., quinidine). Large U waves may be associated with increased risk of torsade de pointes (see Fig. 14.17).

Severe hyperkalemia must be considered immediately in any patient with an unexplained wide QRS complex, particularly if P waves are not apparent. Delay in making this diagnosis can be fatal because severe hyperkalemia may lead to asystole and cardiac arrest while the clinician is waiting for the laboratory report (see Figs. 10.5 and 10.6).

Review

Like most clinical tests, the ECG yields both *false-positive* and *false-negative* diagnoses. For example, not all Q waves indicate myocardial infarction (MI) and not all patients with actual MI show diagnostic ECG changes. A normal or nondiagnostic ECG also does not exclude left ventricular hypertrophy, right ventricular hypertrophy, intermittent life-threatening brady-arrhythmias or tachyarrhythmias, pulmonary embolism, or pericarditis. Despite limitations in sensitivity and specificity, the ECG can provide valuable information in a wide range of clinical situations. Besides its obvious utility in assisting cardiac diagnosis, the ECG may also help in evaluating some major medical problems (e.g., syncope, coma, weakness, shock).

Questions

1. Which arrhythmias can lead to syncope (fainting)?

True or false (Questions 2 and 3)

2. A normal exercise tolerance test excludes significant coronary disease.
3. The more false-positive results associated with a particular test, the less sensitive the test is.

Pacemakers: A Brief Introduction

This chapter provides a brief overview of an important aspect of clinical electrocardiography—electronic cardiac pacemakers. Particular emphasis is placed on the different types of pacemakers, major indications for pacemaking, and recognition of pacemaker malfunction.

Definitions

A pacemaker is a battery-powered device designed to electrically stimulate the heart. This device is used primarily when a patient's own heart rate is excessively slow.* A pacemaker has two major components: a battery that serves as the power source and wire electrodes that are attached to the heart chamber(s) being stimulated.

Pacemakers are either *temporary* or *permanent (implanted).* With temporary pacemakers the pacing wire is connected to a battery outside the body. With long-term implanted pacemakers, the battery is inserted subcutaneously, usually under the chest wall. With both types the pacemaker wire is usually threaded through a vein into the right ventricular cavity so that the pacemaker electrode can stimulate the endocardium of the right ventricle (Fig. 20.1). Occasionally an *epicardial* pacemaker wire is used. This wire is sewn directly into the epicardium of the left or right ventricle, and the battery is implanted under the skin of the abdomen. Atrial pacing can also be

performed. Many patients benefit from a *dual-chamber* pacemaker in which electrodes are placed in both the right atrium and right ventricle.

Pacemaker ECG Patterns

When a ventricular pacemaker fires, it produces a sharp vertical deflection (pacemaker spike) followed by a QRS complex (representing depolarization of the ventricle). Can you predict what the ECG shows with a functioning right ventricular pacemaker? The ECG should show a left bundle branch block (LBBB) pattern (see Fig. 7.8). Recall that the pacemaker is stimulating the right ventricle initially and therefore left ventricular depolarization is delayed.

Typical pacemaker tracings are shown in Figs. 7.8 and 20.2. The vertical line preceding each QRS complex is the pacemaker spike. This sharp deflection is followed by a wide QRS complex with an LBBB morphology (QS in lead V_1 and wide R wave in lead V_6). What pattern would you predict with an epicardial pacemaker stimulating the left ventricle? It would be a right bundle branch block pattern.

An atrial pacemaker produces a spike followed by a P wave (Fig. 20.3).

Pacemaker Batteries

A variety of battery units can be used to power implanted pacemakers. Early pacemaker batteries

---

*See the discussion of bradyarrhythmias in Chapter 18.

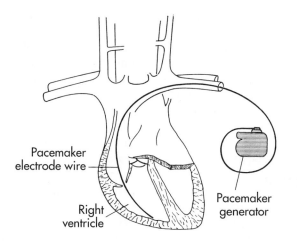

Fig. 20.1 Implanted pacemaker generator (battery) with a wire electrode inserted through the left subclavian vein into the right ventricle.

Ventricular (VVI) Pacemaker

Fig. 20.2 Pacemaker beats. The first P-QRS cycle is from a normal sinus beat. It is followed by four pacemaker beats. Notice the pacemaker spike *(S)* preceding each paced beat. Pacemaker beats are wide and resemble bundle branch block beats. Because this type of pacemaker senses and paces only in the right ventricle and is inhibited by the intrinsic QRS complexes, it is termed a VVI unit. (See Appendix at the end of this chapter.)

Atrial Pacemaker

Fig. 20.3 With the pacemaker electrode placed in the right atrium, a pacemaker spike *(A)* is seen before each *P* wave. The *QRS* complex is normal because the ventricle is not being electronically paced.

used mercury-zinc cells. However, because of their relatively short life span, these units were supplanted by lithium batteries, which may last 5 or more years. As the power cell of a conventional pacemaker wears out, the pacemaker rate usually starts to slow.

Ventricular Pacing: Fixed-Rate and Demand Pacemakers

The two modes of pacemaker function are *fixed rate* and *demand*. A fixed-rate pacemaker is one that fires at a specific preset rate, regardless of the patient's own heart rate. The earliest pacemakers were fixed-rate devices. Contemporary pacemakers are demand units. A demand pacemaker literally functions "on demand" (i.e., only when the patient's heart rate falls below a preset value). Therefore, a demand pacemaker has two distinct aspects: (1) a *sensing* mechanism designed so that the pacemaker is inhibited when the patient's own heart rate is adequate, and (2) a *pacing* mechanism designed to trigger the pacemaker when no

intrinsic QRS complexes occur within a predetermined period. By contrast, fixed-rate pacemakers lack a sensing mechanism.

Demand units can be temporarily converted to fixed-rate mode by placing a special magnet on the chest wall over the battery. The magnet test is routinely performed when the pacemaker rate is being checked. Present-day demand-type pacemakers are also "programmable." This means that the pacing rate can be adjusted once a pacemaker is implanted. Adjustment of rate is accomplished by placing a special telemetry device on the chest wall to allow communication with the pacemaker.

Demand ventricular pacemakers usually are QRS (R wave) inhibited. They emit pulses only when the spontaneous heart rate falls below the escape rate of the pacemaker (e.g., 70 beats/min) (Fig. 20.4). They do not emit pulses when the patient's spontaneous heart rate is faster than the escape rate of the pacemaker. Each time a QRS-inhibited pacemaker senses a spontaneous QRS complex, formation of a pacemaker pulse is inhibited. Therefore these pacemakers show pacemaker

Fig. 20.4 A ventricular demand (QRS-inhibited) pacemaker emits an electronic pulse only when the intrinsic heart rate falls below the escape rate of the pacemaker.

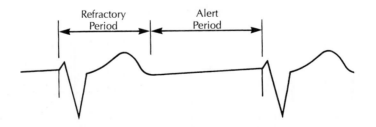

Fig. 20.5 During the refractory period a ventricular demand pacemaker does not sense any electrical activity. The refractory period is followed by the alert period. If no QRS complex is sensed by the end of the alert period, the pacemaker emits an escape pulse.

spikes only when the spontaneous heart rate is slower than the escape rate of the pacemaker. The spikes appear before each QRS complex.

The QRS-inhibited pacemaker also has a *refractory* period (e.g., 0.4 second) that begins whenever the pacemaker senses a QRS complex or emits a pulse (Fig. 20.5). During the refractory period the pacemaker cannot sense another R wave. However, if spontaneous ventricular beats or ventricular premature complexes occur during the refractory period, they are not inhibited but appear on the ECG.

The refractory period is followed by an *alert* period, during which the pacemaker can sense an R wave. If no QRS complex is sensed by the end of the alert period, the pacemaker emits another pulse (Fig. 20.5). However, if a spontaneous QRS complex occurs, the pacemaker is recycled into another refractory period and then into another alert period.

Dual-Chamber Pacing

In dual-chamber pacemakers, electrodes are inserted into both the right atrium and right ventricle. With most models, the circuitry permits sensing and pacing in both chambers. Thus the atrial lead is able to sense the patient's intrinsic P waves and stimulates the atrium when the atrial rate becomes too slow. The circuitry is designed to allow for a physiologic delay between atrial and ventricular stimulation. This *atrioventricular (AV) delay* (interval between the atrial and ventricular pacemaker spikes) is analogous to the PR interval seen in normal conduction.

With the type of dual-chamber pacemaker that allows for both atrial sensing and pacing and ventricular sensing and pacing, a variety of ECG patterns may be seen, depending on the patient's intrinsic electrical activity. A schematic of these pacemaker patterns appears in Fig. 20.6.

Dual-chamber pacing is helpful in maintaining physiologic timing between atrial and ventricular systole. When ventricular pacing alone is used, this physiologic timing is lost. In some patients the loss of timed atrial contractions causes a marked reduction in cardiac output. Dual-chamber pacing produces a significant improvement in the cardiac performance of these individuals. In selected patients, dual-chamber pacing may allow a physiologic increase in ventricular rate during exercise. For example, consider the patient with complete heart block and underlying sinus rhythm whose

Dual-Chamber (DDD) Pacemaker Functions

A. Atrial sensing Ventricular pacing

B. Atrial pacing Ventricular pacing

C. Atrial pacing Ventricular sensing

D. Atrial and ventricular sensing

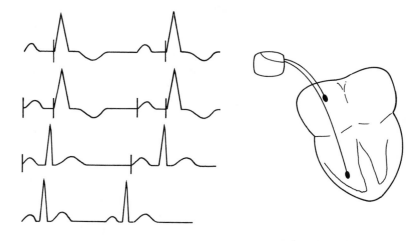

Fig. 20.6 Dual-chamber (DDD) pacemakers sense and pace in both atria and ventricles. The pacemaker emits a stimulus (spike) whenever a native P wave or QRS complex is not sensed within some programmed time interval.

ventricular rate with a ventricular pacemaker is constant (e.g., 72 beats/min) regardless of the atrial (P wave) rate. With a dual-chamber pacemaker the ventricular rate can increase in tandem with the sinus rate during exercise, further increasing cardiac output. Atrial sensing or pacing is obviously of no use in patients with chronic atrial fibrillation or atrial flutter.

Programmability

In the early days of cardiac pacing the pacemaker rate was not adjustable once the unit had been inserted. A major advance was the introduction of programmable pacemakers, in which the pacemaker rate could be externally changed.*

In addition to rate, many other parameters can be externally programmed in modern pacemakers. These parameters include the voltage of the pacemaker discharge, the sensitivity of the electrode to the intrinsic beats, the pacemaker refractory period, and the duration of the pacemaker spike.†

Indications for Cardiac Pacing

IMPLANTED (PERMANENT) PACEMAKERS

The major reason for implanting a pacemaker is the presence of a symptomatic bradyarrhythmia. However, electronic pacemakers may be indicated for numerous other conditions, including syncope, light-headedness, weakness, or congestive failure caused by complete heart block, second-degree AV block, marked sinus bradycardia or sinus pauses (sick sinus syndrome), slow junctional rhythms, or atrial fibrillation or flutter with an excessively slow ventricular response.

Pacemaker functions have also been incorporated in new generations of implantable cardioverter defibrillator devices (see Chapter 14).

---

*Contemporary *rate-responsive pacemakers* are designed with special sensors to detect muscle activity, breathing or other variables that correlate with increased activity. The pacing rate automatically increases with exercise to accommodate the need for increased cardiac output.

†Multiprogrammable pacemakers are discussed in more detail in texts cited in the Bibliography.

TEMPORARY PACEMAKERS

Temporary pacemakers may be *transvenous* or *transcutaneous*. With transvenous pacemakers the battery is connected to a pacing electrode that has been threaded through a vein into the right ventricle. With transcutaneous temporary pacing, specially designed electrodes are pasted on the chest wall. Although this technique is not successful in all patients and may cause some discomfort, it may be useful in certain critical circumstances when transvenous pacing is not available (see Chapter 17).

Temporary pacemakers are often employed during cardiac emergencies (e.g., myocardial infarction [MI]) when an extremely slow heart rate occurs. For example, they may be used immediately after open-heart surgery or during cardiac arrest (see Chapter 17) when the ECG shows asystole or a slow escape rhythm that does not respond to drug therapy. Occasionally, temporary pacemakers are needed in patients with digitalis or other drug toxicity that is causing profound bradycardia.

As noted, temporary or permanent pacemakers are usually employed when the heart rate is too slow. Rarely a pacemaker is implanted to treat a tachyarrhythmia (e.g., ventricular tachycardia). The use of temporary pacing to treat atrial flutter is mentioned in Chapter 13.

Pacemaker Malfunction

Pacemaker malfunctions occur when either the sensing or pacing function is impaired. For example, when the pacemaker battery runs down, the pacing rate generally slows and *failure to sense or pace* may also occur. Failure to sense can be diagnosed by observing pacemaker spikes despite the patient's own adequate rate (Fig. 20.7). The two most common causes of failure to sense (without actual battery failure) are dislodgment of the pacemaker wire and excessive fibrosis around the tip of the pacing wire.

Pacemaker malfunction can also result from *failure to pace*. This problem is diagnosed by observing pacemaker spikes without subsequent QRS complexes (failure to "capture") (Fig. 20.8) or by

Pacemaker Malfunction: Failure to Sense

Monitor

Fig. 20.7 Notice that after the first two paced complexes, a series of sinus beats with a prolonged PR interval is seen. Failure of the pacemaker unit to sense these intrinsic QRS complexes leads to inappropriate pacemaker spikes (●), which sometimes fall on T waves. Three of these spikes do not capture the ventricle because they occur during the refractory period of the cardiac cycle. (Adapted from Conover MH: *Understanding electrocardiography,* ed 4, St Louis, 1996, Mosby.)

Pacemaker Malfunction: Failure to Sense and Capture

Monitor

Fig. 20.8 Notice that beats 1, 3, and 4 show pacemaker spikes *(s)* and normally paced wide QRS complexes and T waves. The remaining beats show only pacemaker spikes without capture. (*R* represents the patient's slow spontaneous QRS complexes, which the pacemaker also fails to sense.)

Pacemaker Malfunction: Failure to Pace

Fig. 20.9 The underlying rhythm is second degree (2:1) atrioventricular block. Despite a slow heart rate, the pacemaker fails to function. (*P,* P waves.)

finding no pacemaker spikes even though the patient has an excessively slow heart rate (Fig. 20.9). Failure to pace can also be caused by dislodgment of the pacemaker wire or by fibrosis around the tip of the pacing wire. In such cases, pacemaker spikes occur without associated QRS complexes. In other cases (particularly with a broken electrode wire, a

short-circuit in the pacing circuit, electrical interference from the muscles of the chest wall, or battery failure), failure to pace occurs without any pacemaker spike.

Pacemaker malfunction in patients with temporary pacemakers should always prompt an immediate search for loose connections between the battery and the pacing wire, a faulty battery, or a dislodged wire.

Complications of Pacemaker Therapy

Pacemakers are not without potential harm. Therefore careful thought should be given before a temporary or particularly a permanent pacemaker is inserted. Infection may occur at the pacemaker site. The electrode may perforate the ventricular wall. The pacemaker itself may cause serious arrhythmias. For example, dual-chamber pacemakers may facilitate runs of supraventricular tachycardia ("endless loop" arrhythmias). Occasionally a pacemaker also paces the muscles of the chest wall or the diaphragm, resulting in patient discomfort.

Diagnosis of Myocardial Infarction with Pacemakers

The ECG diagnosis of MI may be difficult or impossible when all the QRS complexes are paced. With a right ventricular electrode the ECG shows an LBBB configuration. As described in Chapter 8, LBBB generally masks both the QRS and the ST-T changes of MI. Therefore, unless you see spontaneous QRS-T complexes, you may not be able to diagnose acute or prior MI based on the ECG alone.

Finally, pacemakers may also produce ECG changes simulating MI. Following periods of ventricular pacing, the ECG may show deep T wave inversions in the nonpaced beats. These *postpacemaker T wave inversions* can be mistaken for primary ischemic ST-T changes.

Appendix: Pacemaker Code

A three-position pacemaker code is often used to describe a particular pacemaker's functions and mode of response. As shown in Table 20.1, the letter in the first position indicates the chamber(s) being paced—the *atrium (A), ventricle (V),* or *both (D).* The letter in the second position indicates the chamber(s) where sensing occurs—again the atrium (A), ventricle (V), or both (D). Finally, the letter in the third position refers to the mode of response of the pacemaker—*triggered (T), inhibited (I),* or *dual (D).*

Thus a VVI unit is identified as a single-chamber pacemaker that both paces (V) and senses (V) exclusively in the *ventricle* and is *inhibited* (I) by the patient's own QRS complexes.

The most versatile pacemakers are the DDD units. These are dual-chamber pacemakers that can pace the atrium or ventricle (D) and sense in the atrium or ventricle (D). In addition, the mode of response is dual (D). Consequently, atrial pacing can be inhibited by the patient's P waves, and a ventricular pacer spike is triggered by the patient's P waves if a native QRS complex does not appear within a preset time because of atrioventricular block.

The basic three-letter pacemaker code has been expanded to five letters, reflecting rapid advances in pacemaker electronics over the past decade or so. The fourth letter indicates the *programming* features of the pacemaker, including rate responsiveness (R). (See the text discussion of programmability.) Thus a pacemaker that paces and senses just in the right ventricle and has rate-responsive capabilities is designated VVI-R. The fifth letter indicates *special antiarrhythmic features* that are available in certain pacemakers. Further discussion of these technical areas lies beyond the scope of this brief introduction.

Position	Category	Letters used
	Table 20.1 Three-Position Pacemaker Code	
I	Chamber(s) paced	
	Ventricle	V
	Atrium	A
	Dual (atrium and ventricle)	D
	None	O
II	Chamber(s) sensed	
	Ventricle	V
	Atrium	A
	Dual (atrium and ventricle)	D
	None	O
III	Mode of response(s) to sensing	
	Triggered	T
	Inhibited	I
	Dual (triggered and inhibited)*	D
	None	O

*Dual mode of response refers to dual-chamber pacemakers in which atrial pacing may be inhibited by the patient's own P waves and a ventricular spike may be inhibited by the patient's P wave if atrioventricular block is present. A single-chamber (VVI) pacemaker and a dual-chamber (DDD) pacemaker are depicted schematically below.

VVI   DDD

✪ Sensing + Pacing

Review

Pacemakers are battery-powered devices used to stimulate the heart electrically, particularly when a patient's own heart rate is excessively slow. When the pacemaker wire is attached to the right ventricular endocardium, the ECG shows a left bundle branch block pattern because of delayed left ventricular stimulation. Each QRS complex is preceded by a pacemaker spike. Cardiac pacing can be done in a *fixed-rate* or *demand* mode. Demand pacemakers are inhibited when the heart rate is faster than the escape rate of the pacemaker.

A temporary pacemaker is a unit with an external battery. Temporary pacing wires can be inserted during cardiac emergencies (e.g., cardiac arrest caused by asystole or myocardial infarction [MI] complicated by high-degree heart block or sinus arrest). An implanted permanent pacemaker, in which the battery is inserted subcutaneously (usually in the chest wall) is indicated for patients with symptomatic second- or third-degree atrioventricular block or other major bradyarrhythmias (e.g., sinus arrest or slow junctional escape rhythm) leading to inadequate cardiac output.

Dual-chamber (atrial and ventricular) pacemakers were developed to maintain physiologic timing between atrial and ventricular contractions, thereby increasing cardiac output.

When the pacemaker battery starts to run down, the pacemaker rate slows. Dislodgment of the pacemaker wire or excessive fibrosis around the tip of the wire can cause failure to sense or failure to pace. Pacing failure in permanent units can also be caused by electrode fracture, short circuits, or electrical interference from skeletal muscles.

Pacemakers may obscure the ECG diagnosis of MI. Conversely, after electronic pacing of the ventricles, deep noninfarctional T wave inversions may appear in spontaneous QRS complexes *(postpacemaker T wave pattern)*.

Questions

1. Which of the following is the major indication for a *permanent* pacemaker?
   a. History of multiple prior myocardial infarctions
   b. Symptomatic bradyarrhythmia
   c. Digitalis toxicity
   d. Ventricular bigeminy
   e. Paroxysmal supraventricular tachycardia
2. What does the following rhythm strip show?
   a. Failure to sense
   b. Failure to pace
   c. Normal pacemaker function with a ventricular premature beat
   d. Failure to sense and pace

3. What is shown in the following rhythm strip?

21

How to Interpret an ECG

*T*he fundamentals of the normal ECG were discussed in Part 1 of this book, and the major abnormal patterns and arrhythmias have been described thus far in Part 2. Drawing on those concepts and information, this chapter provides a systematic approach to ECG interpretation.

ECG Interpretation

Accurate interpretation of ECGs requires thoroughness and care. Therefore you must develop a systematic method of reading ECGs that is applied in every case. Many of the most common mistakes are errors of omission, specifically the failure to note certain subtle but critical findings. For example, overlooking a short PR interval may cause you to miss the important Wolff-Parkinson-White pattern. Marked prolongation of the QT interval, a potential precursor of torsade de pointes (see Chapter 14) and sudden cardiac death (see Chapter 17), sometimes goes unnoticed. These and other common pitfalls in ECG diagnosis are reviewed in Chapter 19.

ECG FEATURES TO ANALYZE

On every ECG, 14 features should be analyzed. These features are listed in the accompanying box and discussed in the following sections.

Standardization and Technical Features

Make sure that the electrocardiograph has been properly calibrated so that the standardization mark is 10 mm tall (1 mV = 10 mm) (see Chap-

ter 2).* Also check for limb lead reversal (see Chapter 19) and ECG artifacts (discussed later in this chapter).

Heart Rate

Calculate the heart rate (see Chapter 2). If the rate is faster than 100 beats/min, a tachycardia is present. A rate slower than 60 beats/min means that a bradycardia is present.

Be particularly careful not to overlook hidden P waves. For example, these waves may be present in some cases of second- or third-degree atrioventricular (AV) block, atrial tachycardia (AT) with block, or blocked atrial premature beats (APBs). Also, whenever the ventricular rate is about 150 per minute, always consider the possibility of atrial flutter because the flutter waves may mimic the P waves of AT or sinus tachycardia.

Rhythm

The rhythm is usually one of the following: (1) normal sinus rhythm (or a sinus variant such as sinus bradycardia or tachycardia), (2) sinus rhythm with extra (ectopic) beats such as APBs or ventricular premature beats (VPBs), or (3) an entirely ectopic (nonsinus) mechanism such as atrial fibrillation or flutter, ventricular tachycardia, or an AV junctional escape rhythm.

---

*In special cases the ECG may be intentionally recorded at one-half standardization (1 mV = 5 mm) or two-times normal standardization (1 mV = 20 mm).

Features to Analyze on Every ECG

Standardization (calibration) and technical quality
Heart rate
Rhythm
PR interval
P wave size
QRS width (interval)
QT interval
QRS voltage
Mean QRS electrical axis
R wave progression in chest leads
Abnormal Q waves
ST segments
T waves
U waves

PR Interval

The normal PR interval (measured from the beginning of the P wave to the beginning of the QRS complex) is 0.12 to 0.2 second. A uniformly prolonged PR interval is often referred to as *first-degree AV block* (see Chapter 15). A short PR interval with sinus rhythm and with a wide QRS complex and a delta wave is seen in the Wolff-Parkinson-White pattern. By contrast, a short PR interval with retrograde P waves (negative in lead II) generally indicates an ectopic (atrial or AV junctional) pacemaker.

P Wave Size

Normally the P wave does not exceed 2.5 mm in amplitude and is less than 3 mm wide in all leads. Tall, peaked P waves may be a sign of right atrial overload (P pulmonale). Wide P waves are seen with left atrial abnormality.

QRS Width (Interval)

Normally the QRS width is 0.1 second (100 msec) or less in all leads. The differential diagnosis of a wide QRS complex is described in Chapter 10.

QT Interval

A prolonged QT interval may be a clue to electrolyte disturbances (hypocalcemia or hypokalemia), drug effects (quinidine, procainamide, amiodarone, or sotalol), or myocardial ischemia (usually with prominent T wave inversions). Shortened QT intervals are seen with hypercalcemia and digitalis effect.

QRS Voltage

Look for signs of right or left ventricular hypertrophy (see Chapter 6). Remember that thin-chested people and young adults frequently show tall voltage without left ventricular hypertrophy (LVH). Do not forget about low voltage, which may result from pericardial effusion or pleural effusion, hypothyroidism, emphysema, obesity, myocardial disease, or other factors (see Chapter 22).

Mean QRS Electrical Axis

Estimate the mean QRS axis in the frontal plane. Decide by inspection whether the axis is normal (between $-30°$ and $+100°$) or whether left or right axis deviation is present (see Fig. 5.13).

R Wave Progression in Chest Leads

Inspect leads V_1 to V_6 to see if the normal increase in the R/S ratio occurs as you move across the chest (see Chapter 4). Poor R wave progression (small or absent R waves in leads V_1 to V_3)* may be a sign of myocardial infarction (MI), but it may also be seen with altered lead placement, LVH, chronic lung disease, left bundle branch block, and other conditions in the absence of infarction.

Abnormal Q Waves

Prominent Q waves in leads II, III, and aV_F may indicate inferior wall infarction. Prominent Q waves in the anterior leads (I, aV_L, and V_1 to V_6) may indicate anterior wall infarction (see Chapter 8).

ST Segments

Look for abnormal ST segment elevations or depressions.

---

*The term *reversed R wave progression* is used to describe abnormally tall R waves in lead V_1 that progressively decrease in amplitude. This pattern may occur with a number of conditions, including right ventricular hypertrophy, posterior (or posterolateral) infarction, and dextrocardia.

T Waves

Inspect the T waves. Normally they are positive in leads with a positive QRS complex. They are also normally positive in leads V_3 to V_6 in adults, negative in lead aV_R, and positive in lead II. The polarity of the T waves in the other extremity leads depends on the QRS electrical axis. (T waves may be normally negative in lead III even in the presence of a vertical QRS axis.)

U Waves

Look for prominent U waves. These waves may be a sign of hypokalemia or drug effect or toxicity (e.g., quinidine).

FORMULATING AN INTERPRETATION

After you have analyzed the 14 ECG features, you should formulate an overall interpretation. The final ECG reading actually consists of two sections:
1. A list of notable findings
2. An interpretive summary that attempts to integrate or explain these findings

For example, the ECG might show a prolonged QT interval and prominent U waves. The interpretation could be "Repolarization abnormalities consistent with drug effect or toxicity (quinidine, procainamide, etc.) or hypokalemia. Clinical correlation suggested." Another ECG might show wide P waves, right axis deviation, and a tall R wave in lead V_1 (see Fig. 19.1). The interpretation could be "Findings consistent with left atrial abnormality (enlargement) and right ventricular hypertrophy. This combination is highly suggestive of mitral stenosis." In yet a third case the interpretation might simply be "Within normal limits."

You should also formulate a statement comparing the present ECG with previous ECGs (when available).

Thus the ECG is analogous to a newspaper account that consists of the hard facts and then the editorial comment. Like the editorialist, the ECG interpreter may sometimes offer suggestions such as "Serial tracings advisable to evaluate possible evolving ischemic T wave changes." Fig. 21.1 illustrates this systematic approach to ECG interpretation.

Every ECG abnormality you identify should summon up a list of differential diagnostic possibilities (see Chapter 22). *You should search for an explanation of every abnormality found.* For example, if the ECG shows sinus tachycardia, you need to find the cause of the arrhythmia. Is it a result of anxiety, hyperthyroidism, congestive heart failure, hypovolemia, sympathomimetic drugs, alcohol withdrawal, or other causes? If you find ventricular tachycardia, what are the diagnostic possibilities? Is it due to MI or some promptly reversible cause such as hypoxemia, digitalis toxicity, toxic effects of another drug, hypokalemia, or hypomagnesemia? If you see signs of LVH, is the likely cause valvular heart disease, hypertensive heart disease, or cardiomyopathy? In this way the interpretation of an ECG becomes an integral part of clinical diagnosis and patient care.

Computerized ECG Interpretations

Computerized ECG systems are now widely used. These systems provide interpretation and storage of ECG records. The computer programs (software) for ECG analysis have become more sophisticated and accurate.

Despite these advances, computer ECG analyses have important limitations and not infrequently are subject to error. Diagnostic errors are most likely with arrhythmias or more complex abnormalities. Therefore computerized interpretations (including measurements of basic ECG intervals and electrical axes) must never be accepted without careful review.

ECG Artifacts

The ECG, like any other electronic recording, is subject to numerous artifacts that may interfere with accurate interpretation. Some of the most common of these are described here.

60-HERTZ (CYCLE) INTERFERENCE

Interference from alternating-current generators produces the characteristic pattern shown in Fig. 21.2. Notice the fine-tooth comb 60-hertz

Fig. 21.1 ECG for interpretation: (1) standardization—10 mm/mV; 25 mm/sec (electronic calibration); (2) heart rate—75 beats/min; (3) rhythm—normal sinus; (4) PR interval—0.16 second; (5) P waves—normal size; (6) QRS width—0.08 second (normal); (7) QT interval—0.4 second (slightly prolonged for rate); (8) QRS voltage—normal; (9) mean QRS axis—about −30° (biphasic QRS complex in lead II with positive QRS complex in lead I); (10) R wave progression in chest leads—early precordial transition with relatively tall R wave in lead V_2; (11) abnormal Q waves—leads II, III, and aV$_F$; (12) ST segments—slightly elevated in leads II, III, aV$_F$, V_4, V_5, and V_6; slightly depressed in leads V_1 and V_2; (13) T waves—inverted in leads II, III, aV$_F$, and V_3 through V_6; and (14) U waves—not prominent. *Impression:* This ECG is consistent with an inferolateral (or inferoposterolateral) wall myocardial infarction of indeterminate age, possibly acute or evolving. *Comment:* The relatively tall R wave in lead V_2 could reflect loss of lateral potentials or actual posterior wall involvement.

Fig. 21.2 Common ECG artifact produced by 60-Hz interference. **A,** Fast oscillations of the baseline. **B,** Same recording without the artifact.

(Hz) artifacts. You can usually eliminate 60-Hz interference by switching the electrocardiograph plug to a different outlet or turning off other electrical appliances in the room.

MUSCLE TREMOR

Involuntary muscle tremor (e.g., parkinsonism) can produce undulations in the baseline that may be mistaken for atrial flutter or fibrillation (Fig. 21.3).

WANDERING BASELINE

Upward or downward movement of the baseline may produce spurious ST segment elevations or depressions (Fig. 21.4).

POOR ELECTRODE CONTACT OR PATIENT MOVEMENT

Poor electrode contact or patient movement (Fig. 21.5) can produce artifactual deflections in

Fig. 21.3 Common ECG artifact produced by muscle tremor. **A,** Wavy baseline simulating atrial flutter. **B,** Same recording without the artifact, showing normal P waves.

Fig. 21.4 Wandering baseline resulting from patient movement or loose electrode contact.

Fig. 21.5 Deflections simulating ventricular premature beats, produced by patient movement. An artifact produced by 60-Hz interference is also present.

the baseline that may obscure the underlying pattern or be mistaken for abnormal beats.

IMPROPER STANDARDIZATION

The electrocardiograph, as mentioned, should be standardized before each tracing so that a 1-mV pulse produces a square wave 10 mm high (see Fig. 2.5). Failure to standardize properly results in complexes that are either spuriously low or spuriously high. Furthermore, most electrocardiographs are equipped with half-standardization and double-standardization settings. Unintentional recording of an ECG on either of these settings also results in misleading low or high voltage.

Review

The following 14 points should be evaluated on every ECG: standardization, heart rate, rhythm, PR interval, P wave size, QRS width (interval), QT interval, QRS voltage, mean QRS axis, R wave progression in chest leads, abnormal Q waves, ST segments, T waves, and U waves. Any ECG abnormality should be related to the clinical status of the patient.

Computer interpretations of ECGs are subject to error and must be carefully reviewed. The ECG can also be affected by numerous artifacts, including 60-Hz interference, patient movement, poor electrode contact, and muscle tremor.

ECG Differential Diagnoses: A Quick Review

This chapter presents 15 boxes that review selected aspects of ECG differential diagnosis for easy reference. For the most part the boxes recap topics covered in this book. However, some advanced topics are briefly mentioned, with additional discussion available in texts cited in the Bibliography.

Low-Voltage QRS Complexes

1. Artifact: unrecognized standardization of ECG at one-half usual gain (i.e., 1 mV = 5 mm)
2. Normal variant (also seen in pregnancy and obesity)
3. Pericardial tamponade (usually with sinus tachycardia)
4. Pleural effusions
5. Chronic obstructive pulmonary disease
6. Extensive myocardial infarction
7. Myxedema (usually with sinus bradycardia—"low and slow")
8. Cardiac infiltration or replacement (especially cardiac amyloid)
9. Cardiomyopathy (dilation, usually with diffuse fibrosis)
10. Left pneumothorax (mid-left chest leads)

Wide QRS Complex

   I. Intrinsic intraventricular delay*
     A. Left bundle branch block and variants
     B. Right bundle branch block and variants
     C. Other nonspecific patterns of intraventricular delay
  II. Extrinsic ("toxic") intraventricular delay
     A. Hyperkalemia
     B. Drugs: class I antiarrhythmic drugs and related agents (e.g., tricyclic antidepressants and phenothiazines)
 III. Ventricular beats: premature, escape, or paced
 IV. Ventricular preexcitation: Wolff-Parkinson-White pattern and variants

*Bundle branch block patterns may occur transiently. Note also that a spuriously wide QRS complex occurs if the ECG is unintentionally recorded at fast paper speeds (50 or 100 mm/sec).

Right Axis Deviation

   I. Artifact: left-right arm electrode reversal (look for negative P wave and negative QRS complex in lead I)
  II. Normal variant
 III. Dextrocardia
 IV. Right ventricular overload
     A. Acute (e.g., pulmonary embolus)
     B. Chronic
       1. Chronic obstructive pulmonary disease
       2. Any cause of right ventricular hypertrophy (e.g., pulmonic stenosis or primary pulmonary hypertension)
  V. Lateral wall myocardial infarction
 VI. Left posterior hemiblock (exclude all other causes of right axis deviation)

QT Prolongation (Long QT Syndromes)

I. Acquired long QT syndrome
  A. Electrolyte abnormalities
    1. Hypocalcemia
    2. Hypokalemia
    3. Hypomagnesemia
  B. Drugs
    1. Class I or III antiarrhythmic agents (e.g., quinidine, procainamide, disopyramide, sotalol, and amiodarone)
    2. Psychotropic agents (e.g., phenothiazines, tricyclic antidepressants, tetracyclic agents, and haloperidol)
    3. Others: terfenadine, bepridil, certain antibiotics (e.g., erythromycin and pentamidine), probucol, and cisapride (in high doses)
  C. Myocardial ischemia or infarction (with deep T wave inversions)
  D. Cerebrovascular injury
  E. Bradyarrhythmias (especially high-grade atrioventricular heart block)
  F. Systemic hypothermia
  G. Other conditions
    1. Liquid protein diets
    2. Starvation
    3. Myocarditis
    4. Arsenic poisoning
II. Congenital long Q-T syndrome
  A. Romano-Ward syndrome (autosomal dominant)
  B. Jervell and Lange-Nielsen syndrome (autosomal recessive with congenital deafness)

Differential Diagnosis of Q Waves

I. Physiologic or positional factors
  A. Normal-variant septal Q waves
  B. Normal-variant Q waves in leads V_1, V_2, aV_L, III, and aV_F
  C. Left pneumothorax or dextrocardia (loss of lateral R wave progression)
II. Myocardial injury or infiltration
  A. Acute processes
    1. Myocardial ischemia or infarction
    2. Myocarditis
    3. Hyperkalemia
  B. Chronic processes
    1. Myocardial infarction
    2. Idiopathic cardiomyopathy
    3. Myocarditis
    4. Amyloid
    5. Tumor
    6. Sarcoid
III. Ventricular hypertrophy or enlargement
  A. Left ventricular hypertrophy (poor R wave progression*)
  B. Right ventricular hypertrophy (reversed R wave progression†) or poor R wave progression (particularly with chronic obstructive lung disease)
  C. Hypertrophic cardiomyopathy (may simulate anterior, inferior, posterior, or lateral infarcts)
IV. Conduction abnormalities
  A. Left bundle branch block (poor R wave progression*)
  B. Wolff-Parkinson-White patterns

*Small or absent R waves are seen in the right to mid-precordial leads.
†The R wave amplitude decreases progressively from lead V_1 to the mid-lateral precordial leads.

Tall R Wave in Lead V₁

I. Physiologic and positional factors
   A. Misplacement of chest leads
   B. Normal variants
   C. Displacement of heart toward right chest (dextroversion: congenital or acquired)
II. Myocardial injury
   A. Posterior and/or lateral myocardial infarction
   B. Duchenne muscular dystrophy
III. Ventricular enlargement
   A. Right ventricular hypertrophy (usually with right QRS deviation)
   B. Hypertrophic cardiomyopathy
IV. Altered ventricular depolarization
   A. Right ventricular conduction abnormalities
   B. Wolff-Parkinson-White patterns (caused by posterior or lateral wall preexcitation)

ST Segment Elevations

I. Myocardial ischemia or infarction
   A. Noninfarctional transmural ischemia (Prinzmetal's angina pattern)
   B. Acute myocardial infarction
   C. Postmyocardial infarction (ventricular aneurysm pattern)
II. Acute pericarditis
III. Normal variant (early repolarization pattern)
IV. Left ventricular hypertrophy or left bundle branch block (lead V_1-V_2 or V_3 only)
V. Other conditions*
   A. Myocardial injury
      1. Myocarditis (may look like myocardial infarction or pericarditis)
      2. Tumor invasion of ventricles
      3. Trauma to ventricles
   B. Hyperkalemia (leads V_1 and V_2 only)
   C. Hypothermia (J wave or Osborne wave)

*These are rarer causes of ST segment elevations.

ST Segment Depressions

I. Myocardial ischemia or infarction
   A. Acute subendocardial ischemia or non–Q wave myocardial infarction
   B. Reciprocal change with acute transmural ischemia
II. Abnormal noncoronary patterns
   A. Left or right ventricular hypertrophy ("strain" pattern)
   B. Secondary ST-T changes
      1. Left bundle branch block
      2. Right bundle branch block
      3. Wolff-Parkinson-White preexcitation pattern
   C. Drugs (e.g., digitalis)
   D. Metabolic conditions (e.g., hypokalemia)
   E. Miscellaneous conditions (e.g., cardiomyopathy)
III. Physiologic and normal variants*

*With physiologic and normal variants the ST segment depressions are usually less than 1 mm and are seen especially with exertion or hyperventilation.

Prominent T Wave Inversions

I. Primary T wave inversions
  A. Normal variants (e.g., juvenile T wave pattern)
  B. Myocardial ischemia or infarction
  C. Left or right ventricular overload ("strain" pattern)
  D. Cerebrovascular injury
  E. Postpacemaker T wave pattern
  F. Posttachycardia T wave pattern
  G. Miscellaneous conditions
    1. Cardiomyopathies
    2. Pericarditis
    3. Intermittent left bundle branch block
    4. Myocardial tumor
II. Secondary T wave inversions
  A. Left bundle branch block
  B. Right bundle branch block
  C. Wolff-Parkinson-White preexcitation pattern
  D. Ventricular paced beats

Tall Positive T Waves

I. Ischemic causes
  A. Hyperacute phase of myocardial infarction
  B. Acute transient transmural ischemia (Prinzmetal's angina)
  C. Chronic (evolving) phase of myocardial infarction (tall positive T waves reciprocal to primary deep T wave inversions)
II. Nonischemic causes
  A. Normal variants (early repolarization patterns)
  B. Hyperkalemia
  C. Cerebrovascular hemorrhage (more commonly, T wave inversions)
  D. Left ventricular hypertrophy
    1. Right precordial leads, usually in conjunction with left precordial ST depressions and T wave inversions
    2. Left precordial leads, particularly in association with diastolic overload conditions (e.g., aortic or mitral regurgitation)
  E. Left bundle branch block (right precordial leads)
  F. Acute pericarditis (occasionally)

Major Classes of Bradyarrhythmias

I. Sinus bradycardia and its variants, including sinoatrial block
II. Atrioventricular (AV) heart block* or dissociation
  A. Second- or third-degree AV block
  B. Isorhythmic AV dissociation and related variants
III. Junctional (AV nodal) escape rhythms
IV. Atrial fibrillation or flutter with a slow ventricular response
V. Ventricular escape rhythms (idioventricular rhythms)

*Atrioventricular heart block may occur with sinus rhythm or other rhythms (e.g., atrial fibrillation or flutter).

Major Tachyarrhythmias

I. Narrow QRS complex
  A. Sinus tachycardia
  B. Paroxysmal supraventricular tachycardias (PSVTs),* a class of arrhythmias with three major mechanisms:
    1. Atrial tachycardias, including single-focus or multifocal (e.g., multifocal atrial tachycardia [MAT]) variants
    2. AV nodal reentrant tachycardia (AVNRT)
    3. AV reentrant tachycardia (AVRT) involving a bypass tract
  C. Atrial flutter
  D. Atrial fibrillation
II. Wide QRS complex
  A. Ventricular tachycardia (three or more consecutive premature ventricular complexes at a rate of 100 per minute)
  B. Supraventricular tachycardia or atrial fibrillation or flutter, with *aberrant* ventricular conduction usually caused by either of the following:
    1. Bundle branch block
    2. Atrioventricular bypass tract (Wolff-Parkinson-White preexcitation pattern)

*Nonparoxysmal supraventricular tachycardias may also occur, including certain types of junctional tachycardia, as well as *incessant* tachycardias caused by atrial automaticity or a slowly conducting bypass tract.

Causes of Atrial Fibrillation

1. Alcohol ("holiday heart")*
2. Autonomic factors
   a. Sympathetic (occurring during exercise or stress)
   b. Vagotonic (occurring during sleep)
3. Cardiothoracic surgery*
4. Cardiomyopathies or myocarditis*
5. Congenital heart disease
6. Coronary artery disease*
7. Hypertensive heart disease*
8. Idiopathic ("lone" atrial fibrillation)
9. Paroxysmal supraventricular tachycardias or the Wolff-Parkinson-White preexcitation syndrome
10. Pericardial disease (usually chronic)
11. Pulmonary disease (chronic obstructive pulmonary disease)
12. Pulmonary emboli
13. Sick sinus syndrome*
14. Thyrotoxicosis (hyperthyroidism)
15. Valvular heart disease (particularly mitral valve disease)*

*These are among the most common predisposing factors for atrial fibrillation.

Common Arrhythmias in Digitalis Toxicity

I. Bradycardias
   A. Sinus bradycardia, including sinoatrial block
   B. Junctional (nodal) escape rhythms*
   C. Atrioventricular (AV) heart block,* including the following:
      1. Mobitz type I (Wenckebach) AV block
      2. Complete heart block*
II. Tachycardias
   A. Accelerated junctional rhythm* (nonparoxysmal junctional tachycardia)
   B. Atrial tachycardia with block
   C. Ventricular ectopy
      1. Ventricular premature beats
      2. Monomorphic ventricular tachycardia
      3. Bidirectional tachycardia
      4. Ventricular fibrillation

*Junctional rhythms may occur with underlying atrial fibrillation leading to slow or regularized ventricular response. Atrioventricular dissociation without complete heart block may also occur.

Cardiac Arrest: Three Basic ECG Patterns

1. Ventricular tachyarrhythmias
   a. Ventricular fibrillation
   b. Sustained ventricular tachycardia
2. Ventricular standstill (brady-asystolic rhythms)*
3. Electromechanical dissociation*

*The term *pulseless electrical activity* is sometimes used to refer to profound bradycardia or electromechanical dissociation with cardiac arrest.

Part Three

Self-Assessment Problems

The final section of this textbook is a collection of 50 ECGs for review and self-assessment. These unknowns have been selected to challenge students and others who have completed the text or to serve as a stand-alone examination for clinicians who wish to take a board review–type "pretest."

Each question comes with a short case description. (Hopefully helpful clues are sometimes provided.) Students are encouraged to write down their findings and compare their interpretations with the "official" answers given at the end of the section. Each question is worth 2 points. A perfect score is 100!

Questions

....

Life Savers: Stat ECG Diagnoses

The following five patients all have different life-threatening problems that you can diagnose from their ECGs without any further history.

Case 1 60-year-old man

Case 2 50-year-old man

Case 3 68-year-old man

Case 4 75-year-old woman

Case 5 52-year-old man

Triage Tryout

These patients arrive in your office at the same time. Both complain of severe chest pain. One ambulance and one taxicab are available for transporting them to the nearest hospital, which is five miles away. What do you do?

Case 6 50-year-old man with chest pain

Case 7 50-year-old man with chest pain

Four Cases of Mistaken Identity

The following ECGs are commonly incorrectly identified as shown. For each ECG, what is your *correct* diagnosis?

Case 8 "Left bundle branch block or left ventricular hypertrophy with inferior myocardial infarction"

Case 9 "Complete heart block"

Case 10 "Sinus (or ectopic atrial) tachycardia"

Case 11 "Right axis deviation resulting from lateral wall infarction"

Syncopated Rhythms

Both of these patients are complaining of an irregular heartbeat. What are the diagnoses?

Case 12

Case 13

Incomplete Diagnoses of Complete Right Bundle Branch Block

Right bundle branch block was correctly diagnosed in these two patients with chest pain. However, that is only part of the story. What else is going on?

Case 14

Case 15

Morphing P Waves

What subtle arrhythmia is present in this ECG?
Case 16

Tearful Patient

Why is this very healthy female crying? (Clue: Consider QRS duration.)
Case 17

Tricky Business

An ECG is obtained in this 45-year-old man before he undergoes appendectomy. He complains of left lower quadrant pain. The ECG is unchanged from a previous one, at which time the work-up revealed normal heart function. What is the diagnosis?

Case 18

Heart Failure after Myocardial Infarction

Two months after having a myocardial infarction this 75-year-old man presents with rales and S3 gallop. His ECG is unchanged, and cardiac enzymes are negative. What does the ECG show? What did the echocardiogram show?

Case 19

Common Theme

These elderly women have heart failure, and both complain of nausea. What are the two arrhythmias? What is the probable common underlying problem?

Case 20 (Clue: Previous ECGs showed atrial fibrillation with a rapid rate.)

Case 21 (Clue: Double-check leads II and V₁.)

Drug Dilemma

This ECG (from a patient with normal electrolytes) is most consistent with therapy using which of the following drugs:
- a. Digoxin
- b. Captopril
- c. Amiodarone
- d. Metoprolol
- e. Verapamil
- f. None of the above

Case 22

Narrowed-Down Differential Diagnoses

The following patients both have narrowed heart valves. One has mitral stenosis, and the other has pulmonic stenosis. Can you tell which is which?

Case 23

Case 24

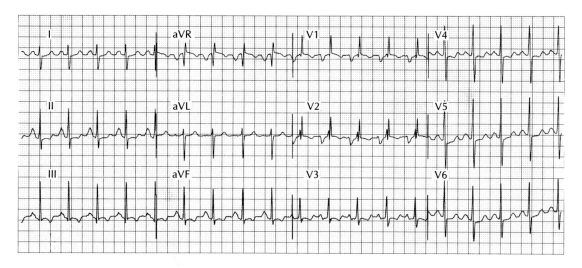

Pause for Thought

A 72-year-old woman has intermittent light-headedness. What does the ECG lead show?

Case 25

Monitor lead

Look-Alike Tachycardias

The following patients both complain of a fast heartbeat. One has atrial flutter with 2:1 block. The other has paroxysmal supraventricular tachycardia (PSVT) due to atrioventricular nodal reentrant tachycardia (AVNRT). Can you tell which is which?

Case 26

Case 27

Silent History

A 75-year-old man has an ECG before undergoing cataract surgery. He denies previous cardiac problems. What does his ECG show?

Case 28

Three Patients with Recurrent Syncope

Case 29   21-year-old woman on no medications with normal electrolyte
concentrations

Case 30   37-year-old man

Case 31 75-year-old woman

Heartburn

This 52-year-old man has indigestion, nausea, and an irregular pulse. What is the rhythm? What is the underlying problem?

Case 32

Hidden P Wave ST-ories

Can you diagnose these two arrhythmias?

Case 33

Case 34

Myocardial Infarction Simulator

This 46-year-old man has chest pain and dyspnea. Initially, he was thought to have had a myocardial infarction. What alternative, life-threatening diagnosis would account for all these findings?

Case 35

Irregular Behavior

The following highly irregular rhythms are often confused. What is the arrhythmia in each case?

Case 36

Case 37

Quick Changes

These two rhythm strips show underlying sinus rhythm with abrupt changes in cardiac electrical activity and intermittent wide QRS complexes. What are the diagnoses?

Case 38

Case 39

Missing Bifocals

A middle-aged cardiologist left his bifocals at home and missed the following diagnosis. (Clue: see arrow.)

Case 40

Long and Short of It

Both of these patients have mental status changes. (Clue: The key to their treatable diagnoses relates to the beginning of the ST segment.)

Case 41 30-year-old woman

Case 42 65-year-old man

Pacemaker Plus

This 78-year-old man has a VVI pacemaker for complete heart block. He comes into the office with shortness of breath and evidence of pulmonary edema. In addition to the expected pacemaker pattern, what does his ECG show?

Case 43

ECG/Coronary Arteriogram Matchup

Which ECG goes best with which story for these four middle-aged men?

Case 44 This man had chest pain 3 days ago. His creatine kinase level is now normal. He has an occluded large left circumflex coronary artery and a severe inferoposterolateral wall motion abnormality.

Case 45 This man has had chest pain for the past 4 hours. His creatine kinase level is 800 U/L (normal: less than 200 U/L). He has three-vessel coronary disease with 80% to 90% proximal stenoses and anterior wall hypokinesis.

Case 46 This man had chest pain 1 month ago, but his creatine kinase level is now normal. Currently he is complaining of dyspnea. He has an occluded proximal left anterior descending coronary artery with an anterior wall aneurysm.

Case 47 This man has had chest pain for 12 hours with a normal creatine kinase level. His coronary arteries and ventricular wall motion are normal.

A

B

10 mm/mv; 25 mm/sec

C

D

Calculations Lead to Diagnosis

A 40-year-old woman complains about feeling weak. She is not taking any medication. Based on the ECG, what laboratory values do you want checked?

Case 48

Interest-Piquing T Waves

But that's not all. (Clues: QRS voltage, P waves, and QT_c.) What underlying condition explains all findings?

Case 49

Fitting Finale

Case 50

Answers to Self-Assessment Problems

Case 1 Severe hyperkalemia. Note the markedly prolonged PR interval and widened QRS complex.

Case 2 Hyperacute phase of anterior wall myocardial infarction. Note the marked ST elevations in leads V_1 through V_6, I, and aV_L, with reciprocal ST depressions in leads III and aV_F. Q waves are present in leads V_3 through V_6. Also note left axis deviation with possible prior inferior wall infarction.

Case 3 Sustained monomorphic ventricular tachycardia. Note the wide-complex tachycardia (QRS duration up to 0.20 second) with a wide R wave in lead V_1, a QS wave in lead V_6, and extreme axis deviation.

Case 4 Sinus rhythm with complete (third-degree) heart block. Note the idioventricular (or very slow junctional) rhythm at about 33 beats/min.

Case 5 Sinus tachycardia with *electrical alternans*. This combination is highly specific for pericardial effusion with tamponade.

Case 6 Acute pericarditis. Note the *diffuse* ST elevations (leads I, II, III, aV_F, and V_3 through V_6) with PR segment deviations (up in lead aV_R, down in leads V_4, V_5, and V_6). This patient gets the taxi.

Case 7 Acute anterior myocardial infarction. ST elevations are *localized* to leads V_1, V_2, V_3, I, and aV_L, with poor R wave progression in leads V_1, V_2, and V_3. In addition, note the *reciprocal* ST depressions in leads II, III, and aV_R. This patient needs an ambulance *immediately*.

Case 8 Wolff-Parkinson-White pattern. Note the triad of short PR intervals, wide QRS complexes, and delta waves (i.e., slurring of the early part of the QRS complexes in leads I, aV_L, V_1, V_2, etc.).

Case 9 Sinus rhythm with isorhythmic atrioventricular dissociation.

Case 10 Atrial flutter with 2:1 block.

Case 11 Left-right arm lead reversal, which accounts for the negative P waves and negative QRS complexes in lead I.

Case 12 Sinus rhythm with Wenckebach-type atrioventricular block.

Case 13 Atrial tachycardia at 150 beats/min with variable block.

Case 14 Right bundle branch block with acute anterior Q wave myocardial infarction. Note the Q waves in leads V_1, V_2, and V_3, with ST elevations in leads V_1 through V_5 and aV_L.

Case 15 Right bundle branch block with anterior subendocardial ischemia. Note the ST depressions in leads V_2, V_3, and V_4.

Case 16 Wandering atrial pacemaker.

Case 17 Normal (and hungry) neonate. Note the very narrow QRS complex (about 0.06 second) with a rightward axis, tall R wave in lead V_1, and fast sinus rate (125 beats/min). All of these findings are appropriate for the patient's age (see Chapter 10).

Case 18 Dextrocardia with situs inversus. Note the apparently reversed limb and chest leads. This patient has a normal heart (right side of chest) and an inflamed appendix (left side of abdomen).

Case 19 Sinus rhythm with prolonged PR interval. The ECG shows left atrial abnormality, left ventricular hypertrophy, and right bundle branch block. Q waves and ST elevations are seen in leads V_1 through V_5, I, and aV_L. The findings are consistent with left ventricular aneurysm, which was confirmed with echocardiography.

Case 20 Atrial fibrillation with a *slow* and at times *regularized* ventricular response should make you suspect digitalis toxicity. ST-T changes are consistent with digitalis toxicity or ischemia, in particular.

Case 21 Atrial tachycardia with 2:1 block. (A very subtle "extra" P wave in the ST segment is best seen in leads V_1 and V_2.) An important cause of this arrhythmia is digitalis toxicity. The ECG shows low voltage in the extremity (limb) leads. Because of the poor R wave progression, this patient may have had a previous anterior myocardial infarction. Based on precordial voltage, left ventricular hypertrophy is present. ST-T changes are consistent with digitalis toxicity, ischemia, left ventricular hypertrophy, etc. The theme common to Cases 20 and 21 is *digitalis toxicity*.

Case 22 c. Amiodarone. Note the markedly prolonged QT(U) interval.

Case 23 Mitral stenosis. The ECG shows signs of right ventricular hypertrophy (i.e., relatively tall R waves in lead V_1 with right axis deviation) and left atrial abnormality.

Case 24 Pulmonic stenosis. The ECG shows signs of right ventricular hypertrophy (relatively tall R waves in lead V$_1$ with right axis deviation) and right atrial abnormality.

Case 25 2:1 sinoatrial block causes an entire P-QRS-T cycle to be "dropped." This patient has symptomatic *sick sinus syndrome* and requires a permanent pacemaker.

Case 26 Atrioventricular nodal reentrant tachycardia (AVNRT). In some of the beats, small retrograde P waves (negative in lead II, positive in lead aV$_R$) are visible immediately after the QRS complex, at the very beginning of the ST segment.

Case 27 Atrial flutter with 2:1 conduction. Note the flutter waves at a rate of 300 beats/min (e.g., leads aV$_R$ and aV$_L$).

Case 28 Inferoposterolateral myocardial infarction. Note the Q waves in leads II, III, aV$_F$, V$_5$, and V$_6$, and the tall R waves in leads V$_1$ and V$_2$.

Case 29 Sinus rhythm with a markedly prolonged QT(U) interval (about 0.6 second). This patient has hereditary long QT syndrome. Syncope was caused by recurrent episodes of a *torsade de pointes*–type of ventricular tachycardia.

Case 30 Atrial fibrillation with Wolff-Parkinson-White syndrome. The clue to the diagnosis is the *extremely rapid wide-complex tachycardia* (about 300 beats/min at times) with a very *irregular* rate.

Case 31 Sinus rhythm at 100 beats/min with advanced second-degree atrioventricular block (3:1 conduction pattern). The QRS complexes show a bifascicular block pattern (right bundle branch block and left anterior fascicular block). Evidence of left atrial abnormality and left ventricular hypertrophy is also present.

Case 32 Sinus rhythm at 95 beats/min with a 4:3 Wenckebach atrioventricular block. Note the group beating pattern. This arrhythmia was due to an evolving Q wave inferior myocardial infarction.

Case 33 Junctional rhythm at 60 beats/min. Note the negative P waves "hidden" at the end of the ST segments.

Case 34 Atrial tachycardia with 2:1 block. Note the "hidden" P wave in the ST segments. The atrial rate is 160 beats/min with a ventricular rate of 80 beats/min.

Case 35 Acute cor pulmonale, in this case due to massive pulmonary embolism. Note the sinus tachycardia, S$_1$Q$_{III}$ pattern, poor R wave progression, and prominent anterior T wave inversions, caused here by right ventricular overload ("strain").

Case 36 Multifocal atrial tachycardia (MAT).

Case 37 Atrial fibrillation (AF).

Case 38 Sinus rhythm with intermittent left bundle branch block. First, three sinus beats are conducted with a left bundle branch block pattern; the next three beats occur with a normal QRS complex. Note the rate slowing, which is associated with normalization of the QRS complex. Therefore the left bundle branch block here is related to rate (acceleration- or tachycardia-dependent).

Case 39 Sinus rhythm with transient accelerated idioventricular rhythm.

Case 40 Sinus rhythm with *atrial bigeminy* and blocked atrial premature beats. The arrow points to a subtle P wave from an atrial premature beat. This beat came so early that it cannot conduct through the atrioventricular node, which is still refractory after the previous sinus beat.

Case 41 Hypercalcemia. Note the short QT interval with very abbreviated ST segment; thus the T wave appears to take off right from the end of the QRS complex.

Case 42 Hypothermia. Note the characteristic J (Osborne) waves, best seen in leads V$_3$, V$_4$, and V$_5$.

Case 43 Acute inferolateral myocardial infarction superimposed on a ventricular pacemaker pattern. Note the ST elevations in leads II, III, aV$_F$, V$_5$, and V$_6$, and the reciprocal ST depressions in leads V$_1$, V$_2$, and V$_3$.

Case 44 B. Diffuse ST depressions (except in lead aV$_R$), most marked in the anterior leads. These findings are consistent with non–Q wave myocardial infarction.

Case 45 A. Findings consistent with evolving inferoposterolateral myocardial infarction.

Case 46 C. Q waves and ST elevations consistent with anterior wall myocardial infarction and aneurysm.

Case 47 D. Diffuse ST elevations and characteristic PR segment deviations, diagnostic of acute pericarditis.

Case 48 Hypocalcemia. Calculate the QT$_C$, with QT = 0.48 second and RR = 0.85 second. Hence QT$_C$ = $0.48/\sqrt{0.85}$ = 0.52. The prolonged QT$_C$ here is due to a long ST segment. The T wave is normal. Thus the most likely diagnosis is hypocalcemia. In contrast, hypokalemia generally flattens the T wave and prolongs the QT(U) interval.

Case 49 Note the combination of the tall peaked T waves from *hyperkalemia* with the voltage criteria for left ventricular hypertrophy (LVH). (Left atrial abnormality is also present.) This combination strongly suggests *chronic renal failure*, the most common cause of hyperkalemia. Patients with hyperkalemia typically have hypertension as well, leading to LVH. QT prolongation may also be present in patients with chronic renal failure from concomitant hypocalcemia. The QT interval here is slightly prolonged (0.46 second).

Case 50 Cardiac arrest. The rhythm strip shows sinus rhythm with ST segment depressions that are consistent with *ischemia*, followed by the abrupt onset of *ventricular flutter* degenerating quickly into *ventricular fibrillation*. The treatment is defibrillation/resuscitation.

Answers to Chapter Questions

PART ONE

Basic Principles and Patterns

Chapter 1

1. See Fig. 1.1.
2. An electrocardiogram (ECG) is a graphical record of cardiac electrical activity obtained by means of electrodes placed on the surface of the body.

Chapter 2

1. **a.** 50 beats/min
   b. 150 beats/min
   c. Approximately 170 beats/min. Seventeen QRS cycles occur in 6 seconds. Notice the irregularity of the QRS complexes and the absence of P waves. This rhythm is *atrial fibrillation* (see Chapter 13).
2. **a.** Abnormally wide QRS complex (0.16 second)
   b. Abnormally long PR interval (approximately 0.3 second)
   c. Abnormally long QT interval (0.4 second) for rate. The RR interval measures 0.6 second; therefore the heart rate is 100 beats/min (see Table 2.1). The rate-corrected QT ($QT_C = QT/\sqrt{RR}$) is also prolonged, at 0.52 second ($0.4/\sqrt{0.6}$). Normal is 0.44 second or less.
3. **a.** Prolong the PR interval.
4. **b.** Prolong the QRS interval.
5. **a.** R wave
   b. qRS complex
   c. QS complex
   d. RSR′ complex
   e. QR complex
6. Drugs (quinidine, procainamide, disopyramide, sotalol, amiodarone), electrolyte abnormalities (hypocalcemia, hypokalemia), hypothermia, myocardial infarction

Chapter 3

1. Lead II = lead I + lead III; therefore, according to Einthoven's equation, lead III = lead II − lead I, as shown below:

III

Notice that the voltages of the P wave, QRS complex, and T wave in lead II are equal to the sum of the P, QRS, and T voltages in leads I and III.

2. The voltages in lead II do *not* equal those in leads I and III. The reason is that leads II and III were mislabeled. When you reverse the labels, the voltage in lead II equals the voltages in leads I and III.
3. See Fig. 3.7, *C.*
4. The positive poles of leads aV_R and II point in opposite directions (see Fig. 3.7).

Chapter 4

1. **a.** Yes. The P waves are positive (upright) in lead II and negative in lead aV_R, with a rate of about 75 beats/min.
   b. Electrically vertical. The R waves are most prominent in leads II, III, and aV_F.

c. The transition zone is in lead V_3. Notice that the RS complexes have the R wave approximately equal to the S wave.

d. The PR interval is about 0.16 second. This is within normal range (0.12 to 0.2 second).

e. The QRS width is 0.08 second. This is normal (less than or equal to 0.1 second).

f. Yes.

2. No. Although a P wave appears before each QRS complex, it is negative in lead II. With sinus rhythm the P should be positive (upright) in lead II. Thus in this patient the pacemaker must be outside the sinus node (ectopic), probably in a low atrial focus near the atrioventricular junction. Inverted P waves such as these are called *retrograde* because the atria are depolarized in the opposite direction from normal (i.e., from the bottom to the top rather than from the top [sinus node] to the bottom [atrioventricular junction]; see also Chapters 11 and 12).

Chapter 5

1. The QRS axis is roughly +60°. Notice that the QRS complex in lead aV_L is biphasic. Therefore the mean QRS axis must point at a right angle to −30°. In this case the axis is obviously about +60° because leads II, III, and aV_F are positive. Note that the R wave in lead III is slightly taller than the R wave in lead I. If the axis were exactly +60°, these waves would be equally tall. Thus the axis must be somewhat more positive than +60°, probably around +70°. Estimating the QRS axis to within 10° or 20° is usually quite adequate for clinical diagnosis.

2. *A*, lead II; *B*, lead I; *C*, lead III. *Explanation:* If the mean QRS axis is −30°, the QRS axis is pointed toward lead I (which is at 0°) and away from lead III (which is at +120°). Obviously lead I must be *B* and lead III must be *C*. Lead II is *A*, which is biphasic. The positive pole of lead II is at +60° on the hexaxial diagram. If the mean QRS axis is −30°, lead II must show a biphasic complex because the mean QRS axis is at right angles to that lead.

Chapter 6

1. a. About 75 beats/min

b. The PR interval is prolonged (about 0.22 second) because of first-degree atrioventricular block (see Chapter 15). The P wave in lead II is also abnormally wide and notched (notice the two humps) as a result of left atrial abnormality (enlargement).

Chapter 7

1. See Fig. 7.6.

2. a. 0.12 second.

b. Right bundle branch block

c. Secondary T wave inversions may be seen in the right chest leads with right bundle branch block (see text and answer to Question 4).

3. Left bundle branch block. The PR interval is also prolonged (0.24 second), referred to as *first-degree atrioventricular block*.

4. *Primary* T wave abnormalities are due to actual changes in ventricular repolarization caused, for example, by drugs, ischemia, or electrolyte abnormalities. These abnormalities are independent of changes in the QRS complex. *Secondary* T wave changes, by contrast, are related entirely to alterations in the timing of ventricular depolarization and are seen in conditions in which the QRS complex is wide. For example, with bundle branch block a change in the sequence of depolarization also alters the sequence of repolarization, causing the T wave to point in a direction opposite the last deflection of the QRS complex. Thus with right bundle branch block the T waves are secondarily inverted in leads with an rSR′ configuration (e.g., V_1, V_2, and sometimes V_3). With left bundle branch block the secondary T wave inversions are seen in leads with tall wide R waves (V_5 and V_6). Secondary T wave inversions are also seen with ventricular paced beats (see Fig. 7.8) and the Wolff-Parkinson-White preexcitation pattern (see Fig. 10.20). Sometimes, primary and secondary T wave changes are seen on the same ECG, as when ischemia develops in a patient with a bundle branch block (see Fig. 8.21).

5. True

6. True

7. True

Chapters 8 and 9

1. a. 100 beats/min

b. Yes. In leads II, III, and aV_F, with reciprocal ST depressions in leads V_2 to V_4, I, and aV_L

c. Yes. Best seen in leads III and aV_F

d. Acute inferior wall infarction

2. a. About +90°. Between 80° and 90° is acceptable.

b. No

c. No. Notice the inverted T waves in leads V_2 to V_6, I, and aV_L.

d. Anterior wall infarction, possibly recent or evolving

3. Reciprocally depressed

4. Ventricular aneurysm

5. b. Non–Q wave infarction

6. Marked ST segment depressions. This patient had severe ischemic chest pain with a non–Q wave infarct.

7. The ECG shows a right bundle branch block pattern with an evolving anterior Q wave infarct. With uncomplicated right bundle branch block the right chest leads show an rSR′ pattern. Note that leads V_1, V_2, and V_3 show wide QR waves (0.12 second) because of the anterior Q wave myocardial infarction and right bundle branch block. The ST elevations in leads V_1, V_2, and V_3 and the T wave inversions across the chest leads are consistent with recent or evolving myocardial infarction.

Chapter 10

1. **b.** Early repolarization pattern
   d. Ventricular aneurysm
   g. Pericarditis
2. **a.** Digitalis effect, *B*
   b. Hyperkalemia, *A*
   c. Hypokalemia, *C*
3. **d.** Wolff-Parkinson-White pattern. Notice the diagnostic triad of a wide QRS complex, a short PR interval, and a delta wave (slurred initial portion of the QRS complex). Compare this with Fig. 10.20, which also shows the Wolff-Parkinson-White pattern. These patterns are sometimes mistaken for hypertrophy (tall R waves) or infarction (*pseudoinfarction* Q waves).

PART TWO
Cardiac Rhythm Disturbances
Chapter 11

1. Yes. The P waves are negative in lead aV$_R$ and positive in lead II. Do not be confused by the unusual QRS complexes (positive in lead aV$_R$ and negative in lead II) produced by the abnormal axis deviation. The diagnosis of normal sinus rhythm depends only on the P waves.
2. No. Each QRS complex is preceded by a P wave. However, notice that the P waves are *negative* in lead II. These retrograde P waves indicate an ectopic pacemaker, probably located in a low atrial site near the atrioventricular junction.

Chapter 12

1. The palpitations could be due to occasional atrial premature beats. Notice that the fifth complex is an atrial premature beat (or possibly a junctional premature beat because the P wave is not seen).
2. Junctional escape beat. Notice that it comes after a pause in the normal rhythm and is not preceded by a P wave.
3. **a.** Approximately 210 beats/min. Count the number of QRS complexes in 6 seconds and multiply by 10.
   b. Paroxysmal supraventricular tachycardia. A retrograde P wave may be seen just after the QRS complex, making atrioventricular nodal reentrant tachycardia (AVNRT) the most likely mechanism for the arrhythmia. However, a concealed bypass tract cannot be excluded here.

Chapter 13

1. **a.** About 300 beats/min
   b. About 75 beats/min
   c. Atrial flutter with 4:1 atrioventricular conduction
2. **a.** About 70 beats/min. Count the number of RR cycles in 6 seconds and multiply by 10.
   b. Atrial fibrillation. This is a subtle example because the fibrillatory waves are of very low amplitude. The diagnosis of atrial fibrillation is suspected when an irregular ventricular response is found along with fine wavering of the baseline between QRS complexes.

3. Slower
4. Faster
5. False

Chapter 14

1. Ventricular tachycardia (monomorphic)
2. Torsade de pointes. Notice the changing orientation and amplitude of the QRS complexes. Contrast this with the ECG in Question 1, where all QRS complexes are the same.
3. Hypoxemia, digitalis or other drug toxicity, hypokalemia, hypomagnesemia (see text)
4. Sinus rhythm with ventricular bigeminy

Chapter 15

1. **a.** Sinus rhythm with AV Wenckebach block. Notice the succession of P waves, with increasing PR intervals followed by a dropped (nonconducted) P wave. This pattern leads to "group beating." Blocked premature atrial contractions can also cause group beating, but the nonconducted P wave comes early (before the next sinus P wave is due). The P waves in this example come on time.
2. **a.** 100 beats/min
   b. 42 beats/min
   c. No
   d. Sinus rhythm with complete heart block. Notice that some of the P waves are hidden in QRS complexes or T waves.

Chapter 16

1. Hypokalemia, hypomagnesemia, hypoxemia, acute myocardial infarction, renal failure (Other answers can be found in the text of Chapter 16.)
2. True
3. False
4. False
5. True

Chapter 17

1. No. By definition, patients with electromechanical dissociation have relatively normal electrical activity. The problem is that this electrical activity is not associated with adequate mechanical (pumping) action, because of, for example, diffuse myocardial injury, pericardial tamponade, or severe loss of intravascular volume. A pacemaker would not help in this situation because the patient already has adequate electrical stimulation.
2. **a.** Idioventricular escape rhythm
   b. External cardiac compression artifacts
3. Digitalis (digoxin), epinephrine, cocaine, quinidine (also procainamide, disopyramide, other antiarrhythmic agents)

Chapter 18

1. **a.** Irregular
   b. No. The baseline shows an irregular fibrillatory pattern.
   c. Atrial fibrillation

2. Ventricular tachycardia
3. Paroxysmal supraventricular tachycardia (probably atrioventricular nodal reentrant tachycardia; see Chapter 12)
4. Sinus rhythm with 2:1 AV block, indicated by a sinus rate of about 74 beats/min and a ventricular rate of about 37 beats/min
5. Digitalis toxicity, hyperkalemia, excess beta blocker, excess calcium channel blocker, hypothyroidism

Chapter 19

1. Syncope can be caused by a variety of bradyarrhythmias or tachyarrhythmias, including excessive sinus bradycardia, sinus arrest, atrioventricular (AV) junctional escape rhythms, second- or third-degree AV block, atrial fibrillation with an excessively slow ventricular response, ventricular tachycardia, paroxysmal supraventricular tachycardias (PSVTs), and atrial fibrillation or flutter with a rapid ventricular response.

2. False
3. False. The sensitivity of a test is a measure of how well the test can detect a given abnormality. False-positive results (abnormal results in normal subjects) lower a test's specificity, not its sensitivity.

Chapter 20

1. **b.** Symptomatic bradyarrhythmia
2. **b.** Failure to pace. In this example of intermittent failure to pace, the fourth pacemaker spike is not followed by a QRS complex. The two most common causes of failure to pace (with a pacemaker spike that does not capture) are dislodgment of the electrode wire and fibrosis around the pacing wire tip. In some cases of pacemaker failure, no pacing spikes are seen (see Fig. 20.9).
3. Atrial pacing. Notice that the sharp pacemaker spike before each P wave is followed by a normal QRS complex (see Fig. 20.3).

Bibliography

CHAPTERS 1 TO 7
Basic Concepts and Patterns

Berne RM, Levy MN: *Cardiovascular physiology,* ed 7, St Louis, 1997, Mosby.

Burch GE, dePasquale NP: *A history of electrocardiography,* Chicago, 1964, Year Book.

Dunn MI, Lipman BS: *Lipman-Massie clinical electrocardiography,* ed 8, Chicago, 1989, Year Book.

Goldberger E: *Unipolar lead electrocardiography and vectorcardiography,* ed 3, Philadelphia, 1953, Lea & Febiger.

Goldman MJ: *Principles of clinical electrocardiography,* ed 12, Los Altos, Calif, 1986, Lange.

Mirvis DM: *Electrocardiography: a physiologic approach,* St Louis, 1993, Mosby.

CHAPTERS 8 AND 9
Myocardial Ischemia and Infarction

Froelicher VF: *Exercise and the heart,* ed 3, Chicago, 1993, Year Book.

Goldberger AL: *Myocardial infarction: electrocardiographic differential diagnosis,* ed 4, St Louis, 1991, Mosby.

Schamroth L: *The electrocardiology of coronary artery disease,* Oxford, 1975, Blackwell.

CHAPTER 10
Miscellaneous Patterns

Chou TC, Knilans TK: *Electrocardiography in clinical practice,* ed 4, Orlando, Fla, 1996, Grune & Stratton.

Goldberger AL: A specific ECG triad associated with congestive heart failure, *PACE* 5:593, 1982.

Park MK, Guntheroth WG: *How to read pediatric ECGs,* ed 3, St Louis, 1992, Mosby.

CHAPTERS 11 TO 21
Arrhythmias, Conduction Disturbances, and Pacemakers
General References

Cardiac Arrhythmia Suppression Trial (CAST): Increased mortality due to encainide or flecainide in a randomized trial of arrhythmia suppression after myocardial infarction, *N Engl J Med* 321:406, 1989.

Josephson ME: *Clinical cardiac electrophysiology,* ed 2, Philadelphia, 1992, Lea & Febiger.

Kastor JA: *Arrhythmias,* Philadelphia, 1994, WB Saunders.

Prystowsky FN, Klein GJ: *Cardiac arrhythmias: an integrated approach for the clinician,* New York, 1994, McGraw-Hill.

Rose BD, editor: Arrhythmias and ECG sections. In *UpToDate (CD-ROM),* Wellesley, Mass, 1998, UpToDate.

Zipes D: Cardiac arrhythmias. In Braunwald EB, editor: *Heart disease: a textbook of cardiovascular medicine,* ed 5, Philadelphia, 1997, WB Saunders.

Zipes D, Jalife J: *Cardiac electrophysiology: from cell to bedside,* ed 2, New York, 1995, Grune & Stratton.

Selected Additional References

ECG-SAP: electrocardiography self-assessment program, Bethesda, Md, 1997-1998, American College of Cardiology.

Textbook of advanced cardiac life support. Dallas, 1997, American Heart Association.

Index